The Comprehensive Management of Parkinson's Disease

The Comprehensive Management of Parkinson's Disease

Edited by
Matthew B. Stern, M.D.
and
Howard I. Hurtig, M.D.
Department of Neurology
University of Pennsylvania
and
The Graduate Hospital
Philadelphia

PMA PUBLISHING CORP.
New York

NOTICE: The editors, contributors, and publisher of this work have made every effort to ensure that the drug dosage schedules and/or procedures are accurate and in accord with the standards accepted at the time of publications. Readers are cautioned, however, to check the product information sheet included in the package of each drug they plan to administer. This is particularly important in regard to new or infrequently used drugs. The publisher is not responsible for any errors of fact or omissions in this book.

Library of Congress Cataloging in Publication Data

The Comprehensive management of Parkinson's disease

    Includes index
    1. Parkinsonism.   I. Stern, Matthew B.   II. Hurtig,
Howard I. [DNLM: 1. Parkinson Disnase — therapy.
WL 359 C737]
RC382.C775 1988   616.8'33   88-25405
ISBN 0-89335-311-6
ISBN 0-89335-316-7 (pbk.)

Printed in the United States of America

Contributors

JAMES BENNETT, M.D., PH.D
Assistant Professor
Department of Neurology, Behavioral
  Medicine, Psychiatry and Pharmacology
University of Virginia School of Medicine
Charlottesville, Virginia

ROGER DUVOISIN, M.D.
Professor and Chairman
University of Medicine and Dentistry of
  New Jersey
Robert Wood Johnson Medical School
Director, Neurology Service
Robert Wood Johnson University
  Hospital
New Brunswick, New Jersey

STANLEY FAHN, M.D.
H. Houston Merritt Professor of
  Neurology
Department of Neurology
Columbia University
College of Physicians and Surgeons
New York, New York

CHRISTOPHER GOETZ, M.D.
Associate Professor
Department of Neurological Sciences
Rush Presbyterian/St. Luke's Medical
  Center
Chicago, Illinois

LAWRENCE GOLBE, M.D.
Assistant Professor Neurology
University of Medicine and Dentistry of
  New Jersey
Robert Wood Johnson Medical School
New Brunswick, New Jersey

HOWARD HURTIG, M.D.
Professor of Neurology
University of Pennsylvania
Co-Director, Movement Disorder Center
The Graduate Hospital
Philadelphia, Pennsylvania

HAROLD KLAWANS, M.D.
Professor of Neurological Sciences and
  Pharmacology
Rush Presbyterian/St. Luke's Medical
  Center
Chicago, Illinois

KAREN MARDER, M.D.
Department of Neurology
Columbia University
College of Physicians and Surgeons
New York, New York

C. DAVID MARSDEN, M.D.
Professor of Neurology
University Department of Neurology
National Hospital for Nervous Disease
Queen Square
London, England

RICHARD MAYEUX, M.D.
Associate Professor
Department of Neurology and Psychiatry
Columbia University
College of Physicians and Surgeons
New York, New York

C. WARREN OLANOW, M.D.
Professor of Neurology
Director, Parkinson's Disease Center
University of South Florida
Tampa, Florida

MATTHEW B. STERN, M.D.
Assistant Professor of Neurology
University of Pennsylvania
Co-Director, Movement Disorder Center
The Graduate Hospital
Philadelphia, Pennsylvania

CAROLINE TANNER, M.D.
Associate Professor
Department of Neurological Sciences
Rush Presbyterian/St. Luke's Medical
   Center
Chicago, Illinois

GWYN VERNON, R.N., M.S.
Nurse Coordinator, Movement Disorder
   Center
Department of Neurology
The Graduate Hospital
Philadelphia, Pennsylvania

Contents

Preface

THE TREATMENT OF PARKINSON'S DISEASE (PD) has changed in recent years. While new drugs have been developed, careful observations and longitudinal studies have reshaped our approach to conventional pharmacotherapy with such drugs as levodopa, amantadine, and bromocriptine. We therefore felt that the time was right for a systematic review of the important diagnostic and therapeutic challenges of the last decade.

The book is divided into four sections: Introduction, treatment of early disease, treatment of advanced disease and future considerations. The introductory section includes a chapter on clinical characteristics, differential diagnosis and assessment of parkinsonism. Recognition that the syndrome of parkinsonism is a heterogeneous disorder of diverse etiologies enables the clinician to formulate a rational treatment plan and more accurately predict prognosis. Chapters on the epidemiology and the natural history of Parkinson's disease and the biochemical pharmacology and pathology of Parkinson's disease are included in this section. A clear understanding of the natural course of PD and the structural and chemical changes that occur in the parkinsonian brain are fundamental to clinical mastery of the most complicated aspects of treating this disease.

Section two reviews the management of early PD. Dr. C. David Marsden eloquently simplifies the ongoing dilemma of when to use levodopa—early or late? Experience with dopamine agonists such as bromocriptine has broadened in recent years. The use of bromocriptine in early disease and its potential for deferring or preventing late complications of treatment is reviewed. The comprehensive approach to the parkinsonian patient is discussed in Chapter 6. Successful treatment of PD requires an understanding of both the physical and psychological impact of a chronic disorder on the patient and family. Establishing a strong support network, including the rational use of ancillary health services, forms the foundation from which comprehensive care can be provided.

Within section four are chapters pertaining to the management of advanced disease. Levodopa revolutionized the treatment of PD but has challenged physicians to become more expert in the management of advanced disease and drug-related complications. The clinical features and treatment of these problems, the use of dopamine agonists in advanced PD and the management of behavioral problems (depression, dementia and drug induced psychosis) that so frequently disable the parkinsonian patient are discussed.

The final section of the book is a discussion of the future management of Parkinson's disease by Dr. Stanley Fahn, who has already contributed substantially to our understanding of movement disorders and their treatment. Recent advances in treatment have paved the way for a variety of novel therapeutic strategies that will refine our management of Parkinson's disease in the coming years.

This monograph combines the knowledge and experience of an internationally renowned group of experts in the field of Parkinson's disease with our own experience at the Graduate Hospital Parkinson's Disease and Movement Disorder Center, which was established in 1982 to provide comprehensive care to parkinsonian patients and their families. The goal of the center is to merge the sophisticated understanding of pharmaco- therapeutic strategies with the ability to recognize and address the myriad of difficulties that patients and family members encounter as they accommodate to the limitations of progressive disease. It is in the spirit of comprehensive care that this work was conceived and we dedicate the book to parkinsonians everywhere, whose courage and faith lend strength to our own commitment "to ease the burden and to find the cure."

Matthew B. Stern, M.D.
Howard I. Hurtig, M.D.
Editors

The Comprehensive Management of Parkinson's Disease

I
An Overview

Chapter 1

The Clinical Characteristics of Parkinson's Disease and Parkinsonian Syndromes: Diagnosis and Assessment

Matthew B. Stern

IN 1817, JAMES PARKINSON DESCRIBED the syndrome of "shaking palsy" and the symptoms of the disease that would eventually bear his name [60]. Although *Parkinson's disease* is a distinct clinical entity, *parkinsonism* is a clinical syndrome that can occur in many disease states. The processes and substances capable of producing parkinsonism include specific types of neuronal systems degeneration, dopamine-depleting and dopamine-blocking drugs, toxins, metabolic disorders, and, less commonly, infections, and structural lesions such as strokes and tumors. Clinical parkinsonism must therefore be approached with a differential diagnosis in mind so that a rational diagnostic and therapeutic approach to the patient can be achieved. Moreover, the ability of practitioners to recognize the various *parkinsonian syndromes* will ultimately contribute to a more precise schema of classification and a better understanding of the epidemiology and pathophysiology of parkinsonism.

PARKINSON'S DISEASE

Parkinson's disease accounts for approximately 75% of all cases of parkinsonism. It affects all races, with a slight male predominance [35], and rivals cerebrovascular disease as a leading cause of neurologic disability. Affecting 1% of the population over the age of 55, Parkinson's disease is characterized by its cardinal manifestations of tremor, rigidity, bradykinesia, and postural instability (Table 1.1), response to medication,

3

Table 1.1 Manifestations of Parkinson's Disease

Cardinal Manifestations of Parkinsons Disease

Tremor
Rigidity
Bradykinesia
Postural Instability

Secondary Manifestations of Parkinson's Disease

Incoordination	Edema
Micrographia	Scoliosis
Blurred vision	Kyphosis
Impaired upgaze	Pain and sensory symptoms
Blepharospasm	Seborrhea
Glabellar reflex	Constipation
Dysarthria	Urinary urgency, hesitancy and frequency
Dysphagia reflex	Loss of libido
Sialorrhea	Impotence
Masked facies	Freezing
Hand and foot deformities	Dementia
Dystonia	Depression

---

and specific pathology. Degeneration of the neurons of the substantia nigra and a proliferation of intracytoplasmic inclusions (Lewy bodies) are the distinct pathologic features of this form of parkinsonism.

The onset of Parkinson's disease is often insidious with nonspecific symptoms. Subtle changes in personality and a feeling of malaise or easy fatigability may occur years prior to the more classic clinical manifestations. Mild slowing, changes in handwriting and coordination, a feeling of weakness, or nonspecific pain are frequently attributed to normal aging or may result in time-consuming and costly medical evaluations. As the disease evolves, more typical signs and symptoms emerge.

Tremor

The tremor of Parkinson's disease is the most recognized and classic symptom, and is the presenting complaint in approximately 75% of patients. Tremor generally occurs early in the course of disease, but may never occur in some parkinsonian patients. The most common tremor of

Parkinson's disease occurs at rest with a frequency of 4-5 cycles per second. The tremor can be a to-and-fro motion of a limb, or it can be associated with more complex thumb and digit movements, with alternating opposition of the thumb and fingers (pill-rolling). The tremor is variable and intermittent. It disappears during sleep and increases under stress. It usually begins in the distal part of one arm, subsequently spreads to the ipsilateral leg, and can eventually generalize to involve all limbs as well as the jaw and lower facial muscles. Postural and kinetic tremors can occur in Parkinson's disease, and their presence should not deter the correct diagnosis if associated with other parkinsonian signs. The isolated occurrence of an action tremor (familial tremor, benign essential tremor) should not be confused with Parkinson's disease.

The mechanism of tremor in Parkinson's disease is unknown. Electrophysiologic data demonstrate alternating synchronized firing between agonist and antagonist muscle groups, but the anatomic basis of tremor is controversial. Experimental animals require cerebellar and rubrospinal lesions in addition to nigrostriatal disconnection in order to produce a resting tremor, although it is deafferentation (disinhibition) of the thalamus via basal ganglia and cerebellum that appears to be crucial in producing the typical rest tremor of Parkinson's disease [50]. However, the neurotoxin MPTP (see below) is selectively nigral-toxic and can produce a classic parkinsonian rest tremor [13]. The variability of tremor reflects its complex linkage with neuronal circuits everywhere, as evidenced by its fluctuating severity in response to mood, motor activity, general health, posture, and even time of day.

Rigidity

The rigidity of Parkinson's disease is a form of hypertonicity that is distinguished from other disinhibiting conditions. The continuous hypertonicity of rigidity differs from spasticity, which is characterized by intermittent resistance to passive movement (the clasped-knife phenomenon). Spasticity is associated with hyperreflexia, extensor plantar responses, motor weakness, and a silent electromyogram at rest. Rigidity has none of these features and can be demonstrated electromyographically by continuous muscle activity [34]. The increase in resistance may be smooth (lead pipe), or ratchety (cogwheeling), as in Parkinson's disease. The cogwheeling effect is felt to be due to the superimposed tremor rhythm [21] and can be demonstrated in the limbs or axial muscles. Like the tremor of Parkinson's disease, rigidity can increase with stress.

Bradykinesia

Bradykinesia differs from rigidity in that it reflects slowness of active movement rather than an abnormality of passive movement. Bradykinesia can therefore occur in the absence of rigidity and vice versa. Slowness in initiating movement is characteristics of Parkinson's disease and is associated with facial masking, difficulty rising from a chair, impaired manual dexterity, and difficulty in performing sequential or repetitive motor acts. Patients have difficulty initiating movement and the time required to complete a task is delayed. Although correct muscles are activated and the relationship between agonists and antagonists is appropriate, the initial surge of motor activity is inadequate and movements are fragmented into a series of incremental steps [51].

Loss of Postural Reflexes

Changes in gait and balance are often the major cause of disability in patients with Parkinson's disease. The mildly symptomatic patient with unilateral disease may exhibit only a slight reduction in arm swing when walking and a tendency to drag the leg on the affected side. As the disease evolves, the affected limb is held in a flexed, adducted position, and steps become short and shuffling (festination). Associated arm movements are lost. Turning and initiation of gait, particularly when walking through doorways, may be hampered by sudden freezing (see below) or stutter steps (start or turn hesitation). Normal postural reflex mechanisms are lost, causing stooped posture, tilting of the trunk, and a tendency to fall forward (propulsion) or backward (retropulsion), which can be demonstrated by gently pushing or pulling the patient. The patient appears to be chasing his center of gravity as he propulses, and the tendency to fall becomes prominent. Severe loss of postural reflexes can eventually confine a patient to a wheelchair or bed, resulting in complications of immobility such as pneumonia and thromboembolic phenomena.

SECONDARY MANIFESTATIONS OF PARKINSON'S DISEASE

In addition to the classic signs of tremor, bradykinesia, rigidity, and loss of postural reflexes, there are many other signs and symptoms that can occur at various stages of Parkinson's disease (Table 1.1). Although there is often a prodromal phase of nonspecific symptoms, including joint pains, weakness, depression, and easy fatigability, these subtle symptoms often go unnoticed by the patient because of their minor impact on functional abilities. However, the secondary manifestations that can evolve in the course of Parkinson's disease are potentially disabling—and yet can lead to erroneous diagnoses, thus delaying effective treatment. Those secondary manifestations that typically accompany advanced disease are discussed in more detail in Chapter 7.

Dexerity and Coordination

Subtle impairment in manual dexterity and generalized incoordination can occur in the absence of overt neurologic signs in patients with Parkinson's disease. A decline in athletic abilities, such as a failing tennis serve or increasing golf score, may be the first clue of neurologic impairment. Handwriting becomes small and illegible (micrographia).

Eventually, manual dexterity is affected and routine activities of daily living, such as dressing and shaving, become more burdensome. Buttoning a shirt or manipulating an eating utensil are common areas of functional limitation.

Visual and Bulbar Dysfunction

Visual complaints and ocular findings are common in Parkinson's disease. Patients often complain of blurred vision, although there is no demonstrable abnormality of the visual system. Eye movements are slow and hypometric (cogwheel pursuit) and impairment of upgaze is common. Ocular motility in Parkinson's disease is otherwise normal. Blepharospasm has been observed in Parkinson's disease, as has "apraxia" of eyelid opening [46]. Finally, a glabellar reflex, in which patients are unable to inhibit the blinking response to forehead tapping (Meyerson's sign) is typically seen in parkinsonian patients.

Speech and swallowing can become impaired in Parkinson's disease. The patient with early Parkinson's disease may slur words or experience a diminution in speech volume (hypophonia). With disease progression, speech becomes muffled and monotonic, and there is loss of normal emotional expression (aprosody). Similarly, swallowing dysfunction evolves as a result of pharyngeal akinesia. Excessive drooling (sialorrhea) may be only a nuisance, but dysphagia in advanced Parkinson's disease can result in malnutrition and aspiration pneumonia; swallowing dysfunction, however, is a more common feature of progressive supranuclear palsy and multiple system atrophy (see below). Finally, akinesia of facial muscles results in the expressionless, fixed, vacant stare (masked facies) that is so characteristic of Parkinson's disease.

Musculoskeletal Changes

A variety of musculoskeletal changes occur in Parkinson's disease, particularly hand and foot deformities. A typical parkinsonian hand (striatal hand) includes ulnar deviation with flexion of metacarpophalangeal and distal interphalangeal joints, and hyperextension of the proximal interphalangeal joints. Similar changes occur in the feet, with curling of the toes and extension of the great toe. Additionally, patients can experience painful, "dystonic" cramps that can occur independent of drug therapy.

Abnormal truncal posturing is common in Parkinson's disease. Typically, a mild scoliosis develops. The scoliosis is concave, contralateral to the affected side. With progression of the disease, a kyphoscoliosis evolves, contributing to the severe postural changes that occur with advanced parkinsonism.

Compression neuropathies involving the brachial plexus and proximal radial nerve have also been reported in Parkinson's disease and are generally a consequence of profound immobility [44]. Finally, patients with Parkinson's disease often complain of swelling of the extremities. Leg edema is likely secondary to venous stasis caused by prolonged immobility, as improvement in motor function generally reduces edema.

Pain and Sensory Symptoms

Various types of pain and sensory complaints are common in Parkinson's disease, contrary to classic teaching. Goetz et al. noted pain directly related to parkinsonism in approximately 50% of a random group of parkinsonians [28]. Pain consisted of muscle cramps, stiffness, dystonia, radiculopathy, and arthralgias. In many patients pain was maximal at the height of parkinsonian disability.

Similarly, sensory symptoms occur frequently in Parkinson's disease and are not associated with peripheral nerve disease [41,76]. Numbness, tingling, and burning can occur at any stage of disease, both on and off medication, and have even preceded motor manifestations, thus leading to erroneous diagnoses. Koller noted paresthesias in approximately 40% of his patients, and, although symptoms did not correlate with motor or autonomic signs, sensory complaints commonly occurred on the side of motor dysfunction in hemiparkinsonians [41]. The basal ganglia may have a role in sensory processing [49], and it has been postulated that sensory symptoms in Parkinson's disease arise when the striatal input to sensory centers such as the thalamus is altered [76].

Dermatologic Changes

Seborrheic dermatitis is the typical dermatologic manifestation of Parkinson's disease. The scalp is involved, as are the eyebrows, eyelids, pinnae, nasal folds, axillae, thorax, and the crural folds.

Gastrointestinal and Genitourinary Dysfunction

Bowel and bladder complaints are universal in Parkinson's disease. Impaired colonic motility slows the transit of feces through the colon. Moreover, fluid depletion and immobility enhance the likelihood that constipation will develop. Similarly, bladder dysfunction with urinary urgency, frequency, and hesitancy is common. Both urinary and gastrointestinal symptoms can be aggravated by antiparkinsonism medications (see Chapter 7).

Autonomic Dysfunction

Although autonomic dysfunction is more a feature of multiple system atrophy (see below), autonomic changes do occur in Parkinson's disease [5,27]. In addition to the bowel and bladder symptoms described above, sexual dysfunction, with loss of libido and impotence, is not uncommon. The cause of impaired sexual function in Parkinson's disease is likely multifactorial. The depression that commonly accompanies Parkinson's disease will diminish libido. Motor disability will also hamper sexual performance, as evidenced by the improvement in sexual ability that can occur with drug therapy. Whether there is a specific effect of dopamine deficiency or of basal ganglia dysfunction on sexual function is unknown. Autonomic instability is also manifested by the excessive sweating that can occur in Parkinson's disease independent of drug therapy. Moreover, studies of autonomic parameters in parkinsonian patients (pulse rate, orthostatic blood pressure, response to Valsalva, and cold pressor stimuli) on and off levodopa have shown that the underlying disease is associated with a mild degree of autonomic dysfunction [27].

Freezing

Patients with Parkinson's disease can experience the sudden, involuntary arrest of voluntary movement. Although *freezing* has been considered a feature of the bradykinesia of parkinsonism, it is actually a separate phenomenon that can occur independent of tremor, rigidity, or bradykinesia. Characterized by an inability to initiate movement or carry out repetitive acts such as finger tapping, writing, or speaking, freezing is most disabling

Table 1.2 A Classification of Parkinsonism

I. Primary (idiopathic, lewy body, nigral degeneration)
II. Secondary (symptomatic)
    A. Infectious (post-encephalitic, luetic, Creutzfeldt-Jakob)
    B. Vascular (lacunar state)
    C. Drug-induced (phenothiazines, butyrophenones, reserpine, metaclopramide)
    D. Toxins (MPTP, Manganese, Carbon Disulphide, Cyanide, Carbon Monoxide)
    E. Metabolic
        Wilson's disease
        Hepatocerebral degeneration
        Hallervordan-Spatz disease
        Hypoparathyroidism
    F. Structural
        Brain tumors
        Hydrocephalus (normal pressure hydrocephalus)
        Head trauma
III. Degenerative
    A. Progressive supranuclear palsy
    B. Multiple system atrophy
        Striatonigral degeneration
        Olivopontocerebellar atrophy
        Shy-Drager syndrome
    C. Spinocerebellar-nigral degeneration
    D. Corticonigral degeneration with neuronal achromasia
    E. Parkinson-dementia complex or Guam (with or without motor neuron disease
    F. Parkinsonism with amyotrophy
    G. Senile gait apraxia
    H. Alzheimer's disease

---

when it affects walking. The patient's feet appear glued to the floor, as he is suddenly and unpredictably immobilized, often causing confusion with the on-off effect that complicates long-term levodopa administration (see Chapter 7). Freezing of gait can also resemble senile gait apraxia and the gait disorder of normal pressure hydrocephalus (see below).

The pathophysiology of freezing in parkinsonism is unknown, but one recent study suggests that it represents a disordered formation of rhythm in repetitive movements that results from defective noradrenergic transmission [58]. However, treatment of freezing with norepinephrine precursors has not resulted in consistent improvement [65].

Cognitive Changes in Parkinson's Disease

Depression and dementia will be covered in more detail in Chapter 9, but are introduced here because of the importance of impaired cognition and mood on functional ability. The prevalence of dementia in Parkinson's disease as defined by *DSM III* criteria approximates 20% [11,67], although many patients perform poorly on tests of visuospatial and perceptual motor function [9,53], while language ability is usually spared [26]. Some investigators have therefore considered cognitive impairment in Parkinson's disease to represent a "subcortical dementia" [55]. However, the distinction between a subcortical dementia and cortical dementia is problematic, as the pattern of intellectual decline in the demented parkinsonian is often indistinguishable from the dementia of Alzheimer's disease [54].

Depression is an integral feature of Parkinson's disease although its exact prevalence and etiology remain uncertain. Depression in Parkinson's disease may be endogenous, related to depletion of brain monamines, or may reflect a premorbid parkinsonian personality predisposed to depression [83]. On the other hand, depression in Parkinson's disease may be the reaction to chronic motor disability and comparable to depression in patients with other chronic diseases [29,82]. Regardless, depression is common in Parkinson's disease and it likely has both reactive and endogenous features. Many patients become withdrawn, passive, and inattentive. Their withdrawal from normal social interactions and everyday life leads to isolation and apathy, further contributing to their overall level of dysfunction (see Chapter 6).

PARKINSONIAN SYNDROMES

The term *parkinsonism* is a generic term that describes a clinical syndrome seen in a number of conditions (Table 1.2). *Parkinson's disease* refers to the common, classic disorder. Although some feel that Parkinson's disease can be further subdivided into tremor-predominant and rigid-akinesia-predominant form [6,90], this distinction has not yet been convincingly established. Secondary or symptomatic parkinsonism can be caused by many other pathologic conditions, necessitating a routine search for treatable and reversible etiologies. Recognizing that parkinsonism is a separate nosologic entity forms the basis for establishing prognosis, choice of therapy, and expected response.

INFECTIOUS PARKINSONISM

The most clinically prevalent form of postencephalitic parkinsonism followed the outbreak of encephalitis lethargica [88], which occurred primarily during the 1920s. Parkinsonism developed months to years after the acute infection. This form of parkinsonism accounted for 12% of all parkinsonian patients seen in a large clinic between 1949 and 1964 [35] although postencephalitic parkinsonism is rarely seen today.

The acute phase of encephalitis lethargica was characterized by hypersomnolence, ophthalmoparesis, cranial nerve palsies and an akinetic rigid state. Involuntary movements such as chorea, dystonia, tics and myoclonus occurred early in the course of disease, and psychiatric manifestations, including delirium and hallucinations, were common. Mortality from the acute infection approached 40%, and approximately half of the survivors developed parkinsonism within 5 years.

Postencephalitic parkinsonism differed clinically from Parkinson's disease in some respects. The age of onset of postencephalitic parkinsonism was considerably younger than the typical age group of Parkinson's disease. The parkinsonism progressed slowly and the mental changes, autonomic instability, and involuntary movements of the acute infection often persisted as part of the subsequent parkinsonian syndrome. Moreover, oculogyric crisis, in which the eyes become fixed in one position, was a characteristic feature of postencephalitic parkinsonism. Patients were sensitive to small amounts of levodopa, although the therapeutic approach was otherwise similar to that of Parkinson's disease.

Postencephalitic parkinsonism is characterized pathologically by depigmentation and neuronal loss in the substantia nigra, as in Parkinson's disease. However, Lewy bodies are seen less frequently, and neurofibrillary tangles and gliosis exist throughout the brainstem. There is also neuronal loss in the striatum.

Infectious causes of parkinsonism are otherwise rare, although a parkinsonian syndrome has been reported in association with other viral infections and as a manifestation of neurosyphilis [59]. Moreover, patients with Creutzfeldt-Jakob disease can develop extrapyramidal symptoms that include tremor, rigidity, and bradykinesia [70].

VASCULAR PARKINSONISM

The term *arteriosclerotic parkinsonism* was introduced by Critchley in 1929 [18], and has been used to describe the parkinsonian appearance of patients with widespread cerebrovascular disease, particularly when associated with dementia, pyramidal tract signs, or pseudobulbar palsy. Although a pure arteriosclerotic cause of Parkinson's disease has not been pathologically documented, the terms *vascular* or *arteriosclerotic* parkinsonism have survived for several reasons. First, parkinsonian patients are in an age group at risk for cerebrovascular disease, so that the coexistence of Parkinson's disease and stroke in the same patient is not unusual. Second, patients with extensive cerebrovascular disease may appear bradykinetic, with short, shuffling steps, rigidity, impaired coordination, and other signs resembling Parkinson's disease. Furthermore, parkinsonism has evolved subacutely following bilateral basal ganglia infarction, supporting the concept of stroke induced parkinsonism [84]. However, the stuttering course of cerebrovascular disease and additional signs such as spasticity, hyperreflexia, and extensor plantar responses should rarely cause confusion with Parkinson's disease. It is likely that several of the patients initially described by Critchley, in fact, had other forms of parkinsonism, such as progressive supranuclear palsy or normal pressure hydrocephalus.

DRUG-INDUCED PARKINSONISM

Drug-induced parkinsonism is clinically indistinguishable from Parkinson's disease and accounts for the majority of patients with secondary (symptomatic) parkinsonism [66]. Drugs that induce parkinsonism either deplete catecholamines from their intraneuronal storage sites (reserpine, tetrabenezine), or block striatal dopamine receptors (phenothiazines, thioxanthenes, and butyrophenones). Reserpine is used predominantly as an antihypertensive agent in humans, and it was the discovery of reserpine-induced parkinsonism in animals that provided the initial clue that catecholamine depletion was relevant to the etiology of Parkinson's disease [14]. Most cases of drug-induced parkinsonism occur in patients receiving major tranquilizers for psychiatric disorders or as antiemetics. Among commonly prescribed neuroleptics, medications most likely to cause parkinsonism include trifluoperazine (Stelazine), fluphenazine (Prolixin, Permatil), perphenazine (Trilafon), prochlorperazine (Compazine), and haloperidol (Haldol). Chlorpromazine (Thorazine) and the thioxanthenes are moderately potent, whereas thioridazine (Mellaril) is a less potent inducer of parkinsonism.

Metaclopramide (Reglan) is a nonphenothiazine compound used in a variety of gastrointestinal disorders, such as nausea and gastroesophageal reflux. Like the neuroleptics, metaclopramide can block central dopamine receptors and cause parkinsonism [31]. The occurrence of typical parkinsonian signs and symptoms after weeks or months of metaclopramide therapy has led to the erroneous diagnosis of Parkinson's disease. Metaclopramide should therefore be used on a short-term basis, avoided in parkinsonian patients, and employed with the same caution as are the neuroleptics.

Symptoms of drug-induced parkinsonism usually begin within severals weeks of initiating therapy. Patients complain of difficulty getting out of a chair, and movement becomes slow and methodical. Gait becomes shuffling and unsteady, particularly when walking through doorways and narrow hallways. Typical parkinsonian signs subsequently evolve with tremor, rigidity, and loss of postural reflexes. Drug-induced parkinsonism is more a function of dose and duration of neuroleptic therapy than an idiosyncratic reaction, and symptoms may persist for months after discontinuing the offending medication. Older patients are more susceptible. There is no evidence that neuroleptics cause Parkinson's disease or speed its progression.

Anticholingeric compounds have been used in drug-induced parkinsonism with some success, although stopping the causative medication is the most prudent course whenever possible. It is hoped that newer drugs (e.g., clozapine and sulpiride) as well as drugs that are now being developed will control psychotic behavior with a lower potential for causing untoward extrapyramidal effects.

NEUROTOXINS

MPTP

The first case of parkinsonism following the intravenous injection of MPTP (1-methyl-4-phenyl-1,2,3,6-tetrahydropyridine) was reported in 1979[19]. However, it was not until 1982, when a small epidemic of parkinsonism occurred in drug users in California, that MPTP became a widely known and studied neurotoxin [45]. MPTP is a by-product of meperidine synthesis and selectively destroys nigrostriatal dopamine neurons [12]. The clinical hallmark of MPTP-induced parkinsonism is the acute onset of symptoms that can be indistinguishable from Parkinson's disease. Patients become rapidly bradykinetic, with rigidity, postural instability, expressionless facies, drooling, dysphonia, and tremor. Although the tremor may be a typical parkinsonian resting tremor, a postural tremor usually predominates. Severely affected patients are immobilized, with marked generalized rigidity, profound dysphagia, and muteness. The clinical, pathological and neuropharmacologic similarities between MPTP-induced parkinsonism and Parkinson's disease will provide a useful framework for studying the pathophysiology of Parkinson's disease, the progression of parkinsonism, and the biochemical and behavioral effects of antiparkinsonian medication.

Manganese

Chronic manganese intoxication can result in a clinical syndrome resembling Parkinson's disease, and occurs in manganese miners as well as workers in manganese ore-crushing plants. Intoxication is thought to result from inhalation and gastrointestinal absorption of manganese dust. The onset of toxic symptoms generally occurs after several months of exposure, with the gradual onset of generalized weakness, irritability, and easy fatigability. Mental symptoms include insomnia or hypersomnolence, as well as apathy, and, occasionally, psychotic behavior. Progressive parkinsonism may follow with generalized bradykinesia, incoordination, hypophonic speech with slurring and stuttering, micrographia, and occasional dystonic postures. The gait disturbance of chronic manganism is prominent. Walking becomes awkward and unsteady, and postural instability with propulsion and retropulsion is characteristic. There may be fine tremor of the limbs, and the facial expression is typically expressionless.

The neurologic manifestations of chronic manganism stabilize following removal from exposure, and some symptoms may even improve with time. However, patients remain impaired and, although chelating agents and antiparkinsonian drugs have been used, treatment is generally disappointing [16].

The pathologic features of manganese toxicity are notable for destruction of the basal ganglia, particularly the globus pallidus. Involvement of the substantia nigra is less constant.

Carbon Disulphide

Inhalation of carbon disulphide vapors occurs in numerous industrial and agriculatural settings. It was initially used in manufacturing rubber and has subsequently been used in the production of rayon and cellophane. It has also been used in grain storage. Inhalation of carbon disulphide vapors causes an acute toxic psychosis, and prolonged exposure results in a variety of neurologic signs, including nystagmus, neuropathy, memory impairment, and personality changes. Permanent dementia can also result from persistent exposure. Parkinsonism was observed in a significant percentage of workers exposed to carbon disulphide, described by Lewy [48]. In a study of 22 grain handlers by Peters et al., there was a high incidence of parkinsonism with cogwheel rigidity, tremor (both resting and action) and loss of associated movements [62].

Cyanide

Cyanide is a rapidly acting, potent toxin that causes cellular respiratory failure by inactivating cytochrome oxidase. Survival following ingestion of cyanide is rare, accounting for a limited description of characteristic neurologic sequelae. Nevertheless, a parkinsonian syndrome can occur in survivors of acute cyanide poisoning. In a case reported by Uitti et al., a young man attempting suicide survived acute cyanide ingestion and developed a persistent parkinsonian syndrome characterized by generalized rigidity, slowness of movement, tremors, and severely impaired postural reflexes [85]. At autopsy, the globus pallidus and putamen were atrophic with spongiform degeneration.

Carbon Monoxide

As with cyanide, carbon monoxide poisoning usually occurs in suicide attempts, although it can occur from chronic exposure in workers exposed to high levels, particularly garage mechanics. Chronic exposure results in loss of appetite, headaches, and dizzy spells. Dysarthric speech with personality changes and frank dementia has been associated with prolonged exposure to high levels of carbon monoxide. Acute, severe carbon monoxide poisoning usually results in anoxic encephalopathy; patients are usually comatose, and survivors experience a variety of neurologic sequelae. In addition to mental confusion and speech disturbances, patients can develop focal neurologic signs, with hemiparesis, hyperreflexia, and extensor plantar responses as well as parkinsonism [39]. Clinically, the parkinsonism of carbon monoxide poisoning resembles Parkinson's disease, but there are usually other associated symptoms, such as emotional lability, dementia, and other focal neurologic signs. The neuropathology of carbon monoxide poisoning includes marked pallidal necrosis in addition to other changes typical of cerebral anoxia.

METABOLIC CAUSES OF PARKINSONISM

Wilson's Disease

Wilson's disease is an autosomal recessive disorder of copper metabolism first described in 1912 by Wilson [89]. A deficiency in the copper carrier protein cerulophasmin is a consistent finding in patients with Wilson's disease and although the pathogenesis of this disorder is excessive accumulation of copper in the brain, liver, cornea, and other organs, the exact relationship between ceruloplasmin deficiency and copper deposition is unknown [72]. Although excessive deposition of copper begins in the liver, approximately 40% of patients with Wilson's disease will present with neurologic manifestations, which are confined to the motor system and usually include a variety of abnormal involuntary movements. Tremor is the predominant neurologic symptom in many patients (pseudosclerotic Wilson's disease). Other patients have more rigidity and dystonic contractures (dystonic Wilson's disease), although most patients will have features of both the pseudosclerotic and dystonic form.

The tremors of Wilson's disease are variable. There can be a typically parkinsonian rest tremor, as well as postural and kinetic tremors. "Wing beating" of the arms is the most severe and dramatic tremor characteristic of Wilson's disease. Other extrapyramidal signs include increased muscle tone with both rigidity and dystonia. Facial expression is fixed, with frequent grimacing. Pharyngeal dysfunction causes severe dysarthria and dysphagia. Other signs include excessive drooling; clumsiness and diminished dexterity; an unsteady, staggering gait; rigidity of the mouth, arms, or legs; choriform movements; grand mal seizures; and a variety of psychiatric disorders including dementia, psychoneurosis, manic-depressive or schizophrenic psychosis, bizarre behavior, and anxiety.

As in Parkinson's disease, the motor disability of Wilson's disease is due primarily to basal ganglia dysfunction. However, corticospinal and corticobulbar pathways can be affected. Sensory abnormalities are noticeably absent.

Other characteristics of Wilson's disease include Kayser-Fleischer rings and liver disease. Kayser-Fleischer rings are the opaque or brownish rings that result from deposition of copper in Descemet's membrane of the cornea. Liver involvement can present as an acute hepatitis, chronic hepatitis, or cirrhosis.

The tremors, rigidity, generalized bradykinesia, posturing of the extremities, and fixed facial expression resemble Parkinson's disease, particularly early in the course of Wilson's disease, which usually presents in the second or third decade of life. It is therefore recommended that any patient in this age group presenting with parkinsonism and other movement disorders be evaluated for Wilson's disease. The evaluation of a patient with suspected Wilson's disease should include a slit-lamp examination, hepatocellular enzymes, serum copper and ceruloplasmin levels, and a 24-hour collection of urine for copper. A quantitative analysis of hepatocellular copper by liver biopsy may be necessary to confirm the diagnosis in selected cases when noninvasive studies are inconclusive [73].

Hepatocerebral Degeneration

Hepatocerebral degeneration occurs following multiple bouts of hepatic encephalopathy and resembles Wilson's disease in combining liver disease with a neurologic syndrome in which extrapyramidal symptoms predominate [38,87]. Patients can experience parkinsonian features, with a rest tremor, bradykinesia, rigidity, and progressive incoordination. Other features include dementia, ataxia, and corticospinal tract signs. The association of a progressive extrapyramidal syndrome with liver failure should not cause confusion with Parkinson's disease.

Hallervorden-Spatz Disease

Hallervorden-Spatz disease is considered a metabolic condition because most evidence suggests that it is a systemic metabolic disorder, even though its manifestations are predominantly neurologic [80]. The cases initially described by Hallervorden and Spatz were characterized by childhood onset of progressive dementia with extrapyramidal signs including bradykinesia, rigidity, and hyperkinetic involuntary movements, particularly dystonia [33]. Many subsequent families with the disease have been reported with variable ages of onset and additional features including ataxia, optic atrophy, dysarthria, and seizures. Hallervorden-Spatz disease can present in young adults and has been reported in an adult presenting with typical parkinsonian features [36]. It should therefore be considered in the differential diagnosis of parkinsonism, particularly in juveniles and young adults.

Hallervorden-Spatz disease is inherited as an autosomal recessive disorder. It is characterized pathologically by degeneration of the globus pallidus and substantia nigra, with accumulation of iron pigment and widespread axonal spheroids. Accumulation of iron pigment is not specific for Hallervorden-Spatz disease, but recent evidence favors a metabolic defect in iron and other pigment metabolism as the likely etiology of this disease [36,80].

Parathyroid Disease

Hypoparathyroidism can be associated with calcification of the basal ganglia and with extrapyramidal symptoms, including tremor, rigidity, bradykinesia and other movement disorders, particularly choreoathetosis. Treatment of the underlying parathyroid disease often improves the neurologic symptoms. An extrapyramidal syndrome including parkinsonism also occurs in familial calcification of the basal ganglia [57]. On the other hand, basal ganglia calcifications are often an incidental finding on skull radiographs or CT scans.

Finally, Fahr described an adult with calcification of striatal vessels [25], and the term *Fahr's disease* has inappropriately been used in cases of basal ganglia calcification of uncertain cause.

STRUCTURAL CAUSES OF PARKINSONISM

Tumors

Although brain tumors are an uncommon cause of parkinsonism, they are included in the differential diagnosis of parkinsonism because of the numerous published case reports. Van Eck reviewed 49 cases of parkinsonism resulting predominantly from gliomas and meningiomas [86]. Direct compression or infiltration of the basal ganglia and interruption of striatal afferent fibers from either the cortex or midbrain are mechanisms by which structural lesions might cause parkinsonism.

Hydrocephalus

Hydrocephalus is associated with a gait disorder and other signs that resemble parkinsonism. Hydrocephalus resulting in elevated intracranial pressure eventually causes headache and altered consciousness, and is rarely misdiagnosed as Parkinson's disease. However, symptomatic hydrocephalus with normal pressure is now a well-recognized entity. The syndrome of normal-pressure hydrocephalus (NPH) was introduced by Hakim and Adams [32] and is now recognized as a potentially reversible cause of progressive dementia, urinary incontinence, and a gait disorder. The gait disorder of hydrocephalus generally evolves prior to the dementia. Steps become short, with a normal or slightly increased base, shuffling, and a tendency of freeze. Even though this type of gait impairment may represent a unique disturbance in the cortical control of ambulation [40], the similarity to the parkinsonian gait is notable. Patients with NPH often appear bradykinetic and may have rigidity, expressionless facies, postural instability, and dementia, thus resembling Parkinson's disease. Tremor is not a feature of NPH.

Patients suspected of having NPH are often subjected to a variety of diagnostic procedures, including CT scans, isotope cisternography, and cerebrospinal fluid infusion tests, although the importance of these diagnostic studies has been challenged. Peterson et al. studied 45 patients with NPH and concluded that clinical presentation and the short duration of symptoms are the most important features of diagnosing NPH and predicting response to ventricular shunting, which carried a significant morbidity in their patients [63]. As in other causes of parkinsonism, the physician must depend heavily on clinical skills to formulate a rational diagnosis and treatment plan.

Head Trauma

Head trauma can cause parkinsonism, as evidenced by the chronic encephalopathy of boxers (punch-drunk syndrome). First reported by Martland in 1928 [52], a variety of clinical syndromes occurring in boxers are now recognized, with mixed patterns of pyramidal, extrapyramidal and cerebellar dysfunction [15]. Early symptoms may be noticed while the boxer is still fighting, and include mild slowing with incoordination, dysequilibrium, and subtle personality changes. Subsequently, more overt cognitive dysfunction evolves and may be associated with slurred speech, tremor, bradykinesia, cogwheel rigidity, and a stooped, festinating gait (pugilistic parkinsonism). Cerebellar signs are also common with intention tremor and ataxia, and pyramidal tract signs with spasticity and pathologic reflexes have been observed. CT scan findings in boxer's encephalopathy include a cavum septum pellucidum and cerebral atrophy. Neuropathologic studies have demonstrated cerebellar damage, widespread neurofibrillary tangles, and depigmentation of the substantia nigra [17]. Although the exact mechanism of brain injury from repeated head trauma is unknown, the incidence of neurologic damage in boxers correlates with the number of professional fights, suggesting that the clinical syndrome results from an accumulation of microscopic brain damage secondary to repeated closed, concussive head injuries.

The onset of parkinsonism following a single episode of head trauma without prolonged coma is a more controversial subject with obvious medicolegal implications. Case reports of parkinsonism following head trauma exist in the literature and although some patients may have Parkinson's disease precipitated or exacerbated by head injury, the occurrence of nigral depigmentation and parkinsonism following isolated head trauma has not been convincingly established.

DEGENERATIVE DISORDERS

Several neuronal degenerative disease produce parkinsonism as part of a clinical syndrome that extends beyond the usual signs and symptoms of

Parkinson's disease. The pathology of these disorders likewise localizes to regions in addition to the substantia nigra, and response to antiparkinsonian medication is poor. Ophthalmoparesis, autonomic failure, ataxia, spasticity, and amyotrophy may occur in any combination with parkinsonism as a heterogeneous group of conditions often referred to as *parkinsonism-plus* or *parkinsonism-multiple system atrophy* [30,71]. They include progressive supranuclear palsy (PSP), striatonigral degeneration (SND), olivopontocerebellar atrophy (OCPA), parkinsonism-autonomic failure or Shy-Drager syndrome (SDS), and other more unusual diseases such as spinocerebellar-nigral degeneration, corticodentatonigral degeneration, parkinsonism with amyotrophy, and the parkinsonism- dementia-amyotrophic lateral sclerosis complex of Guam. Alzheimer's disease and senile gait apraxia are also discussed briefly in this section.

The clinical and pathologic boundaries of the multiple system atrophies may be distinct in some (PSP), while blurred in others (SND, OPCA, SDS). The latter three disorders can ususally be recognized as separate clinical entities, although there tends to be a common underlying pathology affecting neurons in the pons, olive, cerebellum, substantia nigra and striatum. The reason for the variability of clinical expression in the face of a homogenous pathology is unknown.

Progressive Supranuclear Palsy (PSP)

Although case reports of PSP appeared in the literature prior to the 1960s, the syndrome of PSP was formally described in 1964 by Steele, Richardson and Olszweski [77]. PSP is now recognized as a common form of drug resistant parkinsonism and, like Parkinson's disease, it has a world wide distribution. Men are affected more often than women.

The disease is characterized by progressive supranuclear ophthalmoparesis (first vertical gaze then horizontal), nuchal dystonia with opisthotonic rigidity of the neck, pseudobulbar palsy with dysphagia and dysarthria, and marked postural instability. Although this constellation of signs and symptoms may seem easily distinguishable from Parkinson's disease, parkinsonian features may predominate in early PSP whereas the characteristic ophthalmoparesis and other manifestations may not appear for several years after onset.

Early symptoms of PSP are often vague as in Parkinson's disease and include mild disequilibrium with slowing, easy fatigability, minor personality changes, and subtle visual symptoms such as blurring or diplopia. With disease progression, walking becomes slow and deliberate with broad-based steps and postural instability. Axial rigidity is more characteristic of PSP than limb rigidity. A peculiar posturing of the neck may evolve in which the head is fixed skyward (nuchal dystonia). Facial expression is fixed and is often associated with deep furrowing of the nasolabial folds, ptosis, blepharospasm and apraxia of eyelid opening. Early complaints referable to evolving ophthalmoparesis include inability to read, write, eat properly, or dress. Downgaze is classically affected early, with progressive impairment of upgaze. Total ophthalmoplegia can occur in advanced stages. A profound dysarthria and dysphagia frequently occur late and are major problems of long-term management. Tremor is rare. Pyramidal signs with brisk reflexes and extensor plantar responses have been observed.

Apathy, depression, irritability and other personality changes are common features of PSP. Furthermore, congitive dysfunction is also frequent although frank dementia is a less constant feature of PSP than previously thought. Slowing of mental processing in PSP has been referred to as a subcortical dementia [3].

PSP can be differentiated from Parkinson's disease if the typical signs are looked for, such as nuchal posture, absence of tremor, ophthalmoparesis, predominantly axial rigidity, and an unsteady gait. In some cases, particularly early in the course of disease when typical signs are missing, the only clue to diagnosis may be the failure of levodopa to relieve symptoms. Although some of the parkinsonian symptoms may transiently improve with antiparkinsonian medications, the response to drugs is never satisfactory, and the disease progresses relentlessly. The neuropathologic features of PSP include neuronal loss and gliosis in the brainstem, diencephalon, globus pallidus, and cerebellum, with neurofibrillary tangles consisting of straight tubules as opposed to the twisted tubules of Alzheimer's disease (see review by Kristensen [43]).

Striatonigral Degeneration (SND)

Striatonigral degeneration was also described as a separate clinical entity in the early 1960s [1]. SND is often clinically indistinguishable from Parkinson's disease but differs in its natural history, response to antiparkinsonian medications, and neuropathology.

As in Parkinson's disease, patients with SND develop rigidity with generalized bradykinesia, masked facies, a shuffling gait, and hypophonic, muffled speech. Swallowing dysfunction evolves as the disease advances. Dystonic postures are observed, as are personality changes such as anxiety

Table 1.3 The Olivopontocerebellar Atrophies (OPCAs)*

Dominantly inherited
  Menzel type
  Schut and Joseph diseases
  With slow saccades and peripheral neuropathy
  With retinal degeneration
  With dementia and extrapyramidal features
  With glycolipiduria
Sporadic and/or recessively inherited
  Dejerine-Thomas type
  With glutamate dehydrogenase deficiency
  With striatal degeneration (multiple system atrophy)
  With progressive autonomic failure

---

*From Duvoisin, RC [24].

and irritability, which may predate the onset of extrapyramidal signs and symptoms. Dementia does not occur in SND, and a typically parkinsonian rest tremor occurs less commonly than in Parkinson's disease. Moreover, SND steadily progresses, with a course lasting approximately 5 years. Antiparkinsonian medications are always tried, although the response to therapy is generally disappointing. These patients virtually never develop levodopa-induced dyskinesias.

The incidence of SND is unknown, but it probably accounts for the majority of parkinsonian patients with primary levodopa failure. One autopsy study of parkinsonian patients found an 8% incidence of SND [81], the pathology of which consists of a characteristic gross brownish discoloration of the putamen, reflecting severe neuronal loss and gliosis, in addition to cell loss and depigmentation of the substantia nigra. Pathologic changes may also be seen in the cerebellum and other brainstem regions, resulting in additional clinical signs, thus overlapping with olivopontocerebellar atrophy and the Shy-Drager syndrome (see below).

Olivopontocerebellar Atrophy (OPCA)

The term *olivopontocerebellar atrophy* describes a gorup of disorders that are characterized clinically by a mixture of cerebellar, brainstem, and extrapyramidal signs and symptoms. The initial cases described in 1900 by Dejerine and Thomas [20] were patients with progressive ataxia beginning in middle age, associated with generalized slowing, loss of coordination, action tremor, and disturbances in ocular motility. Menzel, however, had previously described the pathology of a similar ataxic disorder with a younger age of onset and autosomal dominant mode of inheritance [56]. OPCA has since become recognized as a heterogeneous disorder with variable inheritance, neuropathology, and clinical manifestations. Konigsmark and Weiner attempted to classify the OPCAs based primarily on clinical and genetic features [42]. However, CT scan documentation of brainstem and cerebellar atrophy has enabled the recognition of a wider group of patients with OPCA. Moreover, biochemical abnormalities have been discovered in several types of OPCA [7,64] and await confirmation in follow-up studies. A classification based on current knowledge of the OPCAs has therefore been suggested by Duvoisin [24] although it is likely that this too will be refined in the near future as our understanding of the biochemistry and pathophysiology of OPCA evolves (Table 1.3).

Parkinsonism is now a well recognized component of OPCA. Patients may in fact present with rigidity, resting tremor, bardykinesia, a fixed facial expression, and shuffling gait, typical of Parkinson's disease. Parkinsonism may mask subtle cerebellar signs, and the casual observer will miss the correct diagnosis. The presence of brainstem and cerebellar atrophy on CT scanning and the failure of patients to respond to antiparkinsonian medications are the clues to premortem diagnosis. The neuropathology of OPCA is widespread with neuronal loss in the inferior olives, basal pontine nuclei, and cerebellar cortex. There may be involvement of cranial nerve nuclei, pyramidal tracts, spinocerebellar tracts, and posterior columns. Additionally, involvement of the basal ganglia and autonomic pathways suggests an overlap with striatonigral degeneration and the Shy-Drager syndrome.

Parkinsonism-Autonomic Failure (Shy-Drager Syndrome)

Autonomic failure can occur in isolation, and has been referred to as *Idiopathic Orthostatic Hypotension* or, more appropriately, *Progressive Autonomic Failure*. When autonomic failure accompanies variable neurologic signs and symptoms including parkinsonism, the eponym *Shy-Drager syndrome* has been employed [75], although the separateness of Shy-Drager syndrome as a nosologic entity is controversial (see below). Signs of autonomic failure include orthostatic hypotension, urinary urgency and retention, anhydrosis, and impotence, all of which likely reflect degeneration of the intermediolateral cell columns and autonomic neurons of the sacral cord [79]. Typical parkinsonian signs associated with autonomic failure in the Shy-Drager syndrome include rigidity, masked facies, resting tremor, bradykinesia, and a shuffling gait. Parkinsonian manifestations may respond transiently to antiparkinsonian medication, although the usefulness of dopaminergic agents is limited because of their propensity to induce or aggravate hypotension. Patients may also exhibit ataxia, amyotrophy, and pyramidal tract signs with spasticity, hyper-reflexia, and extensor plantar responses. The combination of cerebellar, extrapyramidal and pyramidal dysfunction links the Shy-Drager syndrome to OPCA, SND, as well as Parkinson's disease. Moreover, the occurrence of gliosis and cell loss in brain regions, common to all these syndromes (the striatum, substantia nigra, inferior olives, pontine nuclei, cerebellum, and autonomic pathways) provides further evidence that these degenerative disorders are related.

OTHER DEGENERATIVE DISORDERS WITH PARKINSONIAN FEATURES

There are several other disorders that deserve mentioning in a discussion of the differential diagnosis of parkinsonism, although they are rarely encountered in clinical practice.

Spinocerebellar-Nigral Degeneration

Spinocerebellar-nigral degeneration was initially described in six members of a family who developed a gait disorder in the 3rd decade of life [8]. With disease progression, there were variable degrees of tremor, rigidity, and bradykinesia, as well as pyramidal tract signs, peripheral neuropathy, amyotrophy, and ataxia. Parkinsonism associated with Friedreich's ataxia has subsequently been reported in families with dominant inheritance [91], and it is therefore accepted as a separate disease entity.

Corticodentatonigral Degeneration with Neuronal Achromasia

Corticodentatonigral degeneration with neuronal achromasia is a rare familial disorder first described by Rebeiz et al. in a family of Irish decent [68]. These patients were affected in adulthood with a progressive gait disorder, bradykinesia, rigidity, dysarthria, vertical ophthalmoparesis, involunatary movements, proprioceptive loss, and pyramidal tract signs. This disorder only superficially resembles Parkinson's disease but can be mistaken for progressive supranuclear palsy and multiple system atrophy. The characteristic neuropathologic findings are achromasia of cortical neuronal cytoplasm and degeneration of pyramidal tracts, dentate nucleus, and substantia nigra.

Parkinsonism-Amyotrophy

Amyotrophy occurs with parkinsonism in a number of settings, suggesting a possible etiologic relationship between motor neuron disease and Parkinson's disease. First, the Chamorro population on Guam has an inordinately high incidence of parkinsonism-dementia and amyotrophic lateral sclerosis (ALS). Patients experience progressive deterioration of cognitive function associated with typical parkinsonism that responds to antiparkinsonian medications. Additionally, most patients have pyramidal tract signs and approximately one third develop ALS with fasciculations and progressive muscular atrophy [69]. Moreover, the neuropathology of ALS and parkinsonism-dementia in Guamanians is similar, suggesting a shared pathogenesis [4]. Second, many patients with multiple system atrophy (SND, OPCA, Shy-Drager syndrome) have anterior horn cell loss at autopsy [79], and motor neuron disease has been reported in patients with Parkinson's disease [10].

SENILE GAIT APRAXIA

The only disorder of gait that has been ascribed to aging is senile gait apraxia. These patients develop an unsteady gait with short, shuffling steps, out of proportion to other neurologic signs. The base of the stride may widen slightly and the feet appear frozen to the ground, particularly when turning. Propulsion, retropulsion, and festination characteristically evolve, thus resembling the parkinsonian gait. Although rigidity can be observed, it is more paratonic than cogwheeling, and other manifestions of Parkinson's disease, such as tremor and bradykinesia, are notably absent. Nevertheless, patients with senile gait apraxia are frequently misdiagnosed as having Parkinson's disease. Predictably, the response to antiparkinsonian medications is poor.

While neurologists have labeled the shuffling, unsteady gait of elderly patients as *apractic,* the term is unsatisfactory. Apraxia implies the loss of previously learned motor abilities and suggests structural brain disease, particularly in the frontal lobes. However, no brain region has been unequivocally implicated as the sole cause of this type of gait disorder [2], nor is aging alone a likely etiology. Senile gait apraxia undoubtedly represents a multifactorial disturbance of frontal lobe and extrapyramidal control of locomotion, although a more satisfactory explanation awaits pathologic and physiologic confirmation.

Table 1.4 Common Pitfalls in Diagnosing Parkinson's Disease

Disorder mistaken for Parkinson's disease	Parkinson's disease because:
Benign essential tremor	Rest, not action tremor, predominates.
Alzheimer's disease	Extrapyramidal signs predominate and predate dementia.
Rheumatoid arthritis	Hand and foot deformities are striatal posturing, not joint deformities.
Syncope or vertebrobasilar insufficiency	Falling is secondary to postural instability, not loss of consciousness.
Hemiparesis (stroke, tumor)	No focal weakness or pathologic reflexes. Typical striatal postures present with cogwheel rigidity, not spasticity.
Myasthenia gravis	Weakness, dysphagia and easy fatigability are manifestations of extrapyramidal dysfunction, associated rigidity and bradykinesia, absence of muscle weakness.

ALZHEIMER'S DISEASE

Alzheimer's disease is included in the differential diagnosis of parkinsonism because of the frequent appearance of extrapyramidal signs and symptoms. Although dementia is the predominant feature of Alzheimer's disease, a stooped posture with a shuffling gait and generalized slowness are common, as are loss of affect and expressionless facies. Cogwheel rigidity has also been demonstrated, but a resting tremor rarely occurs. Recent autopsy studies have, in fact, demonstrated Lewy bodies and loss of pigmented nuclei typical of Parkinson's disease in patients with Alzheimer's disease and extrapyramidal symptoms during life [22,37]. The occurrence of dementia in Parkinson's disease can pose further diagnostic difficulty, and both Alzheimer's and Parkinson's diseases do coincidentally occur [47]. However, cognitive decline in Parkinson's disease generally follows progressive motor dysfunction, and the parkinsonian features of Alzheimer's disease respond poorly, if at all, to antiparkinsonian medication. Nevertheless, the pathologic similarities between Alzheimer's disease and Parkinson's disease have fostered renewed interest in the neurochemistry of cognitive dysfunction [78].

ASSESSING THE PATIENT WITH PARKINSONISM

The correct diagnosis of parkinsonism is crucial in formulating a reasonable therapeutic approach and predicting long-term prognosis. There are no specific laboratory tests diagnostic of Parkinson's disease, so the

Table 1.5 Clues to Diagnosing Parkinsonian Syndromes

Neurologic sign	Suggested diagnoses
Dementia predominates	Alzheimer's disease, NPH, multiinfarct state
Ophthalmoparesis	PSP, multiple-system atrophy
Amyotrophy	Parkinsonism-motor neuron disease, multiple-system atrophy, Creutzfeldt-Jakob disease
Ataxia	OPCA, multiple-system atrophy
Apraxia	NPH, senile gait apraxia
Autonomic failure	multiple-system atrophy (Shy-Drager syndrome)
Peripheral neuropathy	OPCA, multiple-system atrophy, spinocerebellar-nigral degeneration
Pyramidal tract signs	Multi-infarct state, multiple-system atrophy, cervical myelopathy

history and neurologic examination remain the fundamental clinical tools. The major challenges in approaching the patient with suspected parkinsonism include distinguishing changes of normal aging from neurologic disease, differentiating Parkinson's disease from other, unrelated disorders (Table 1.4), and, finally, differentiating Parkinson's disease from other causes of parkinsonism (Table 1.5).

Normal Aging

Normal individuals in their eighth and ninth decade can experience changes resembling early parkinsonism. Mentation, vision, muscle tone, and gait all undergo change in the course of normal aging. The ability to store new information diminishes with age, but the degree of cognitive impairment may not be severe enough to cause serious limitation. Visual changes of older individuals include impaired convergence and upgaze. A mild degree of muscle rigidity can occur, although the increase in resistance parallels the force of passive movement (paratonic rigidity). Aging is associated with a hesitant gait, increased base, and mildly stooped posture, although significant unsteadiness with falling, disequilibrium, and loss of postural reflexes distinguishes neurologic impairment from normal aging. Moreover, the age of onset of Parkinson's disease is more often in the sixth and seventh decades, before the aforementioned changes of normal aging evolve. Finally, other characteristic changes of Parkinson's disease such as tremor and bradykinesia do not appear in the normal, aged individual.

DIAGNOSING PARKINSON'S DISEASE

History

Establishing the onset of symptoms in parkinsonism may be difficult, because vague complaints such as arthralgias, easy fatigability, mild slowing, and depression may appear years prior to more overt neurologic impairment and are recognized as early parkinsonian symptoms only after the classic manifestations evolve. Early signs such as mild bradykinesia, changes in expression, and subtle manual incoordination may go unnoticed, particularly when functional abilities are minimally affected. Patients are often inaccurate when describing the evolution of their disease and will recount symptoms according to their impact on neurologic disability. As a result, patients usually can report the relatively acute onset of symptoms that have been slowing evolving over many years only after they are suddenly unable to function normally.

Nevertheless, the chronology of symptoms is important to establish. Tremor is the first symptom in the majority of patients with Parkinson's disease whereas the early appearance of a gait disorder might suggest one of the parkinson-plus syndromes such as multiple system atrophy or PSP. Similarly, the history of dementia predating the onset of motor symptoms and presenting as the predominant complaint suggests the possibility of Alzheimer's disease, a multi-infarct state, or normal pressure hydrocephalus. If the history reveals a significant degree of autonomic instability such as urinary urgency, constipation, or loss of libido, the physician must be suspicious of the multiple system atrophies; visual complaints such as diplopia may occur early in the course of PSP.

A positive family history of parkinsonism suggests one of the inherited extrapyramidal disorders such as OPCA and is less commonly seen in Parkinson's disease.

A careful drug history as well as exposure to toxins should be elucidated to exclude the possibility of parkinsonism induced by drugs (e.g., phenothiazines) or toxins (e.g., MPTP).

Finally, if a patient has been treated for parkinsonism, the details of his response to medication should be carefully recorded. A favorable response usually indicates Parkinson's disease, whereas failure to respond suggests one of the multiple system atrophies.

THE EXAMINATION

The neurologic examination of patients with suspected parkinsonism should be approached with attention to specific functions relevant to the extrapyramidal system and important in the differential diagnosis of parkinsonism.

Mental Status

The mental-status examination is generally normal in early Parkinson's disease although varying degrees of cognitive impairment do occur with advancing parkinsonism, and neuropsychological testing may reveal mild impairment. If dementia is the predominant feature, Alzheimer's disease or other dementing disorders should be considered.

Speech

Speech can be affected in all of the parkinsonian syndromes. However, the speech of PSP is more dysarthric (pseudobulbar) than the hypophonic speech of Parkinson's disease. Slow, scanning speech is indicative of cerebellar disease and is more typical of OPCA or multiple system atrophy.

Oculomotor System

Ocular motility is normal in Parkinson's disease, with the exception of impaired upgaze and hypometric pursuit movements. Supranuclear paresis of gaze (particularly vertical gaze), which suggests PSP, is manifested by loss of voluntary gaze and by absent optokinetic responses with preservation of oculocephalic reflexes. Gaze paresis, absent saccades, and unstable fixation can also occur in multiple system atrophy.

Motor System

The tremor, rigidity, and bradykinesia of Parkinson's disease are all demonstrable within the motor examination. The presence of a predominantly action tremor that lessens at rest should alert the examiner to the possibility of benign essential tremor, particularly if rigidity, bradykinesia, and other parkinsonian manifestations are absent. An intention tremor as manifested by dysmetria on finger-to-nose testing is a feature of cerebellar disease and not Parkinson's disease. Cogwheel rigidity is demonstrated by rotating a limb and feeling for the "ratchety" pattern of resistance, which can be differentiated from the intermittent resistence of spasticity and paratonia. The presence of focal motor weakness on examination as well as hyperreflexia and extensor plantar responses should not be confused with hemiparkinsonism. The striatal toe that occurs in parkinsonism can resemble an extensor plantar, which is a reflex movement. Finally, lower motor neuron signs such as amyotrophy and loss of reflexes suggests multiple system atrophy, parkinsonism-amyotrophy, or an associated peripheral neuropathy.

Sensory Examination

A peripheral neuropathy is not a feature of Parkinson's disease. However, peripheral neuropathies can occur in OPCA and in the rare disorder of spinocerebellar-nigral degeneration. Patients with Parkinson's disease are as susceptible as anyone to common disorders affecting peripheral nerves, such as diabetes.

Gait

The gait disorder of extrapyramidal dysfunction should be distinguished from ataxia and apraxia. The parkinsonian base is normal or minimally increased, whereas a widened base suggests an ataxic component as occurs in OPCA. Severe postural instability and a wide base occur in PSP, whereas an increased base with short, shuffling steps and freezing occurs in normal pressure hydrocephalus and senile gait apraxia. A spastic gait is stiff-legged with a narrow base and indicates pyramidal tract dysfunction as in a cervical myelopathy (spondylosis) or bilateral cerebral infarcts, both of which are common in older patients.

Autonomic Function

The easiest autonomic parameter to check is orthostatic blood pressure. Blood pressure should be recorded in the supine, sitting, and standing positions. Significant orthostasis unrelated to dopaminergic medication (see Chapter 7) suggests one of the multiple system atrophies and warrants further autonomic testing such as the response to Valsalva or cold pressor stimuli [27].

DIAGNOSTIC STUDIES

Patients with parkinsonism should undergo a general medical examination and routine clinical laboratory studies to assess general health and the presence of any condition that might contribute to the patients' overall level of functioning. Liver function tests as well as calcium and phosphate levels should be included in the metabolic screen, because hepatic dysfunction and hypoparathyroidism are associated with extrapyramidal symptoms.

The neurodiagnostic laboratory can be helpful in evaluating parkinsonism but should be thoughtfully employed. CT scanning is generally not helpful in Parkinson's disease, and is therefore not recommended for patients with typical, bilateral, drug-responsive Parkinson's disease. Hemiparkinsonism can be confused with focal brain disease, such as tumor or infarction, and imaging is recommended. Patients with drug-resistent parkinsonism or atypical signs such as ataxia, severe dementia, ophthalmoparesis, or pyramidal tract signs should also undergo CT scanning to document the presence of cerebrovascular disease, normal pressure hydrocephalus, or brainstem and cerebellar atrophy.

Magnetic-resonance imaging may prove more useful than CT in demonstrating basal ganglia and brainstem disease. Improved resolution of the posterior fossa outlines brainstem structures in more detail. This is especially important in diseases resulting from degeneration of neuronal systems with atrophy of particular brainstem regions such as the multiple system atrophies and PSP. Moreover, magnetic-resonance imaging may provide metabolic information on the water and iron content of the brain. Preliminary studies have shown variable concentrations of iron in the basal ganglia of patients with Parkinson's disease and parkinsonian syndromes [23,61], underscoring the potential application of this imaging technique to the diagnosis of extrapyramidal diseases.

Other neurodiagnostic studies are less useful. Brainstem auditory evoked responses are occasionally helpful when multiple system atrophy is considered, because an abnormal brainstem auditory evoked response reflects brainstem dysfunction between the auditory nucleus and inferior colliculus. A cerebrospinal fluid examination should be performed if the onset of symptoms is acute or subacute and an infectious etiology is considered.

RATING THE PARKINSONIAN PATIENT

The evaluation of the parkinsonian patient must include an assessment of primary and secondary manifestations as well as specific functional abilities and subjective complaints that are prevalent in parkinsonism and relevant to the patient's overall functional capacity. There have been a number of rating scales that have been used to assess and follow patients with Parkinson's disease. Although all the commonly used scales have similar features, there are differences—both in the parkinsonian signs and symptoms that are stressed, as well as the particular scoring system used. Variations in rating scales can therefore account for some of the differences reported in therapeutic trials of antiparkinsonian medications as well as studies of disease progression. The unified rating scale for parkinsonism has therefore been developed (Table 1.6).* This rating scale includes an assessment of the primary and secondary symptoms of the disease, drug-related fluctuations, mentation, activities of daily living [74], and the basic staging system of Hoehn and Yahr [35].

Table 1.7 is the unified rating scale condensed into a useful score sheet that can serve as an easy reference for the practicing physician or nurse. Each sign and symptom is graded on a 0-4 scale, with 4 being most severe. The patient's progress and predominant symptoms can be easily documented and followed over time so that treatment can be adjusted accordingly.

Included in the scale is a measure of *off times*. The evaluator records the average number of hours a patient is functionally off, and whether or not fluctuations are related to dosing schedule (predictable or unpredictable). The emerging pattern of response to medication will guide the physician in choosing the next appropriate course of therapy.

Dyskinesias can also be recorded on the unified rating scale. The duration of involuntary movements as well as the degree of associated disability and pain are scored.

The Schwab and England scale reflects the patient's ability to perform routine activities of daily living [74]. A score of 100% implies total independence whereas diminishing percentages correlate with both slowness in completing routine needs and progressive loss of independence.

Spaces for the Schwab and England score and the Hoehn and Yahr stage are conveniently located at the bottom of page 2 of the score sheet (Table 1.7) to serve as easy reference points, summarizing the patient's overall level of functioning. Comparing these scores over time can provide a simple means of determining disease progression and response to treatment. A unified means of assessing patients will therefore assist the physician in following patients, as well as provide an accurate framework for clinical investigation of disease progression and effectiveness of treatment.

---

* The Unified Parkinson's Disease Rating Scale was developed by a committee established in October 1984. The members of the committee were Drs. Yves Agid, Donald Calne, Roger DuVoisin, Stanley Fahn, Margaret Hoehn, Joseph Jancovic, Harold Klawans, Anthony Lang, Xaviar Lataste, Abe Lieberman, Charles Markham, David Marsden, Urpo Rinne, Gerald Stern, Paul Teychenne and Melvin Yahr.

Table 1.6 Unified Rating Scale for Parkinsonism Version 3.0—February 1987

Definitions of 0-4 Scale

I. Mentation, behavior and mood
1. *Intellectual impairments:*
    0 = None.
    1 = Mild. Consistent forgetfulness with partial recollection of events and no other difficulties.
    2 = Moderate memory loss, with disorientation and moderate difficulty handling complex problems. Mild but definite impairment of function at home with need of occasional prompting.
    3 = Severe memory loss with disorientation for time and often to place. Severe impairment in handling problems.
    4 = Severe memory loss with orientation preserved to person only. Unable to make judgments or solve problems. Requires much help with personal care. Cannot be left alone at all.
2. *Thought disorder* (due to dementia or drug intoxication):
    0 = None.
    1 = Vivid dreaming.
    2 = "Benign" hallucinations with insight retained.
    3 = Occasional to frequent hallucinations or delusions; without insight; could interfere with daily activities.
    4 = Persistent hallucinations, delusions, or florid psychosis. Not able to care for self.
3. *Depression:*
    0 = Not present.
    1 = Periods of sadness or guilt greater than normal, never sustained for days or weeks.
    2 = Sustained depression (1 week or more).
    3 = Sustained depresison with vegetative symptoms (insomnia, anorexia, weight loss, loss of interest).
    4 = Sustained depression with vegatative symptoms and suicidal thoughts or intent.
4. *Motivation/initiative:*
    0 = Normal.
    1 = Less assertive than usual; more passive.
    2 = Loss of initiative or disinterest in elective (nonroutine) activities.
    3 = Loss of initiative or disinterest in day to day (routine) activities.
    4 = Withdrawn, complete loss of motivation.

II. Activities of daily living (determine for "on/off")
5. *Speech:*
    0 = Normal.
    1 = Mildy affected. No difficulty being understood.
    2 = Moderately affected. Sometimes asked to repeat statements.

Table 1.6 Unified Rating Scale for Parkinsonism Version 3.0—February 1987 (cont)

3 = Severely affected. Sometimes asked to repeat statements.

4 = Unintelligible most of the time.

6. *Salivation:*

0 = Normal.

1 = Slight but definite excess of saliva in mouth; may have nightime drooling.

2 = Moderately excessive saliva; may have minimal drooling.

3 = Marked excess of saliva with some drooling.

4 = Marked drooling, requires constant tissue or handkerchief.

7. *Swallowing:*

0 = Normal.

1 = Rare choking.

2 = Occasional choking.

3 = Requires soft food.

4 = Requires NG tube or gastrotomy feeding.

8. *Handwriting:*

0 = Normal.

1 = Slightly slow or small.

2 = Moderately slow or small; all words are legible.

3 = Severely affected; not all words are legible.

4 = The majority of words are not legible.

9. *Cutting food and handling utensils:*

0 = Normal.

1 = Somewhat slow and clumsy, but no help needed.

2 = Can cut most foods, although clumsy and slow; some help needed.

3 = Food must be cut by someone, but can still feed slowly.

4 = Needs to be fed.

10. *Dressing:*

0 = Normal.

1 = Somewhat slow, but no help needed.

2 = Occasional assistance with buttoning, or with getting arms in sleeves.

3 = Considerable help required, but can do some things alone.

4 = Helpless.

11. *Hygiene:*

0 = Normal.

1 = Somewhat slow, but no help needed.

2 = Needs help to shower or bathe; or very slow in hygienic care.

3 = Requires assistance for washing, brushing teeth, combing hair, going to bathroom.

4 = Foley catheter or other mechanical aids.

12. *Turning in bed and adjusting bed clothes:*

0 = Normal.

1 = Somewhat slow and clumsy, but no help needed.

2 = Can turn alone or adjust sheets, but with great difficulty.

3 = Can initiate, but not turn or adjust sheets alone.

Table 1.6 Unified Rating Scale for Parkinsonism Version 3.0—February 1987 (cont)

4 = Helpless.
13. *Falling (unrelated to freezing):*
 0 = None.
 1 = Rare falling.
 2 = Occasionally falls, less than once per day.
 3 = Falls on average of once daily.
 4 = Falls more than once daily.
14. *Freezing when walking:*
 0 = None.
 1 = Rare freezing when walking; may have start-hesitation.
 2 = Occasional freezing when walking.
 3 = Frequent freezing. Occasionally falls from freezing.
 4 = Frequent falls from freezing.
15. *Walking:*
 0 = Normal.
 1 = Mild difficulty. May not swing arms or may tend to drag leg.
 2 = Moderate difficulty, but requires little or no assistance.
 3 = Severe disturbance of walking, requiring assistance.
 4 = Cannot walk at all, even with assistance.
16. *Tremor:*
 0 = Absent.
 1 = Slight and infrequently present.
 2 = Moderate; bothersome to patient.
 3 = Severe; interferes with many activities.
 4 = Marked; interferes with most activities.
17. *Sensory complaints related to parkinsonism:*
 0 = None.
 1 = Occasionally has numbness, tingling, or mild aching.
 2 = Frequently has numbness, tingling, or aching; not distressing.
 3 = Frequent painful sensations.
 4 = Excruciating pain.

III. Motor examination
18. *Speech:*
 0 = Normal.
 1 = Slight loss of expression, diction, and/or volume.
 2 = Monotone, slurred but understandable; moderately impaired.
 3 = Marked impairment, difficult to understand.
 4 = Unintelligible.
19. *Facial expression:*
 0 = Normal.
 1 = Minimal hypomimia, could be normal "poker face".
 2 = Slight but definitely abnormal diminution of facial expression.
 3 = Moderate hypomimia; lips parted some of the time.

Table 1.6 Unified Rating Scale for Parkinsonism Version 3.0—February 1987 (cont)

4 = Masked or fixed facies with severe or complete loss of facial expression; lips parted 1/4 inch or more.

20. *Tremor at rest:*
    0 = Absent.
    1 = Slight and infrequently present.
    2 = Mild in amplitude and persistent. Or moderate in amplitude, but only intermittently present.
    3 = Moderate in amplitude and present most of the time.
    4 = Marked in amplitude and present most of the time.

21. *Action or postural tremor of hands:*
    0 = Absent.
    1 = Slight; present with action.
    2 = Moderate in amplitude, present with action.
    3 = Moderate in amplitude with posture holding as well as action.
    4 = Marked in amplitude; interferes with feeding.

22. *Rigidity* (judged on passive movement of major joints with patient relaxed in sitting position; cogwheeling to be ignored):
    0 = Absent.
    1 = Slight or detectable only when activated by mirror or other movements.
    2 = Mild to moderate.
    3 = Marked, but full range of motion easily achieved.
    4 = Severe, range of motion achieved with difficulty.

23. *Finger taps* (patient taps thumb with index finger in rapid succession with widest amplitude possible, each hand separately):
    0 = Normal.
    1 = Mild slowing and/or reduction in amplitude.
    2 = Moderately impaired. Definite and early fatiguing. May have occasional arrests in movement.
    3 = Severely impaired. Frequent hesitation in initiating movements or arrests in on going movement.
    4 = Can barely perform the task.

24. *Hand movement* (patient opens and closes hands in rapid succession with widest amplitude possible, each hand separately):
    0 = Normal.
    1 = Mild slowing and/or reduction in amplitude.
    2 = Moderately impaired. Definite and early fatiguing. May have occasional arrests in movement.
    3 = Severely impaired. Frequent hesitation in initiating movements or arrests in ongoing movement.
    4 = Can barely perform the task.

25. *Rapid alternating movements of hands* (pronation- supination movements of hands, vertically or horizontally, with as large an amplitude as possible, both hands simultaneouly):
    0 = Normal.

Table 1.6 Unified Rating Scale for Parkinsonism Version 3.0—February 1987 (cont)

---

      1 = Mild slowing and/or reduction in amplitude.

      2 = Moderately impaired. Definite and early fatiguing. May have occasional arrests in movement.

      3 = Severely impaired. Frequent hesitation in initiating movements or arrests in ongoing movement.

      4 = Can barely perform the task.

26.   *Leg agility* (patient taps heel on ground in rapid succession, picking up entire leg; amplitude should be about 3 inches):

      0 = Normal.

      1 = Mild slowing and/or reduction in amplitude.

      2 = Moderately impaired. Definite and early fatiguing. May have occasional arrests in movement.

      3 = Severely impaired. Frequent hesitation in initiating movements or arrests in ongoing movement.

      4 = Can barely perform the task.

27.   *Arising from chair* (patient attempts to arise from a straight-backed wood or metal chair with arms folded across chest).

      0 = Normal.

      1 = Slow; or may need more than one attempt.

      2 = Pushes self up from arms of seat.

      3 = Tends to fall back and may have to try more than one time, but can get up without help.

      4 = Unable to arise without help.

28.   *Posture:*

      0 = Normal erect.

      1 = Not quite erect, slightly stooped posture; could be normal for older person.

      2 = Moderately stooped posture, definitely abnormal; can be slightly leaning to one side.

      3 = Severely stooped posture with kyphosis; can be moderately leaning to one side.

      4 = Marked flexion with extreme abnormality of posture.

29.   *Gait:*

      0 = Normal.

      1 = Walks slowly, may shuffle with short steps, but no festination or propulsion.

      2 = Walks with difficulty, but requires little or no assistance; may have some festination, short steps, or propulsion.

      3 = Severe disturbance of gait, requiring assistance.

      4 = Cannot walk at all, even with assistance.

30.   *Postural stability* (response to sudden posterior displacement produced by pull on shoulders while patient is erect with eyes open and feet slightly apart; patient is prepared):

      0 = Normal.

Table 1.6 Unified Rating Scale for Parkinsonism Version 3.0—February 1987 (cont)

1 = Retropulsion, but recovers unaided.
2 = Absence of postural response; would fall if not caught by examiner.
3 = Very unstable, tends to lose balance spontaneously.
4 = Unable to stand without assistance.

31. *Body bradykinesia and hypokinesia* (combining slowness, hesitancy, decreased armswing, small amplitude, and poverty of movement in general):
0 = None.
1 = Minimal slowness, giving movement a deliberate character; could be normal for some persons. Possibly reduced amplitude.
2 = Mild degree of slowness and poverty of movement that is definitely abnormal. Alternatively, some reduced amplitude.
3 = Moderate slowness, poverty, or small amplitude of movement.
4 = Marked slowness, poverty, or small amplitude of movement.

IV. Complications of therapy (in the past week)
A. Dyskinesias
32. *Duration: What proportion of the waking day are dyskinesias present?* (historical information)
0 = None
1 = 1-25% of day.
2 = 26-50% of day.
3 = 51-75% of day.
4 = 76-100% of day.

33. *Disability: How disabling are the dyskinesias?* (historical information; may be modified by office examination)
0 = Not disabling.
1 = Mildly disabling.
2 = Moderately disabling.
3 = Severely disabling.
4 = Completely disabled.

34. *Painful dyskinesia: How painful are the dyskinesias?*
0 = No painful dyskinesias.
1 = Slight.
2 = Moderate.
3 = Severe.
4 = Marked.

35. *Presence of early morning dystonia* (Historical inforamtion):
0 = No
1 = Yes

B. Clinical fluctuations
36. *Are any "off" periods predicatable as to timing after a dose of medicaiton?*
0 = No
1 = Yes

37. *Are any "off" periods unpredicatable as to timing after a dose of medications?*
0 = No

Table 1.6 Unified Rating Scale for Parkinsonism Version 3.0—February 1987 (cont)

---

       1 = Yes
38. *Do any of the "off" periods come on suddenly, for example over a few seconds?*
       0 = No
       1 = Yes
39. *What proportion of the waking day is the patient "off" on average?*
       0 = None
       1 = 1-25% of day.
       2 = 26-50% of day.
       3 = 51-75% of day.
       4 = 76-100% of day.
C.   Other complications
40. *Does the patient have anorexia, nausea, or vomiting?*
       0 =No
       1 = Yes
41. *Does the patient have any sleep disturbances, for example, insomnia or hypersomnolence?*
       0 = No
       1 = Yes
42. Does the patient have symptomatic orthostasis?
       0 = No
       1 = Yes

Record the patient's blood pressure, pulse and weight on the scoring form.

V. Modified Hoehn and Yahr staging
- Stage 0   = No signs of disease.
- Stage 1   = Unilateral disease.
- Stage 1.5 = Unilateral plus axial involvement.
- Stage 2   = Bilateral disease, without impairment of balance.
- Stage 2.5 = Mild bilateral disease, with recovery on pull test.
- Stage 3   = Mild to moderate bilateral disease; some postural instability; physically independent.
- Stage 4   = Severe disability; still able to walk or stand unassisted.
- Stage 5 = Wheelchair bound or bedridden unless aided.

VI. Schwab and England activities of daily living scale
- 100%—Completely independent. Able to do all chores without slowness, difficulty, or impairment. Essentially normal. Unaware of any difficulty.
- 90%—Completely independent. Able to do all chores with some degree of slowness, difficulty, and impairment. Might take twice as long. Beginning to be aware of difficulty.
- 80%—Completely independent in most chores. Takes twice as long. Conscious of difficulty and slowness.
- 70%—Not completely independent. More difficulty with some chores. Three to four times as long in some. Must spend a large part of the day with chores.
- 60%—Some dependency. Can do most chores, but exceedingly slowly and with much effort. Errors; some impossible.

Table 1.6 Unified Rating Scale for Parkinsonism Version 3.0—February 1987 (cont)

- 50%—More dependent. Help with half, slower, and so forth. Difficulty with everything.
- 40%—Very dependent. Can assist with all chores, but does few alone.
- 30%—With effort, now and then does a few chores alone, or begins alone. Much help needed.
- 20%—Nothing done alone. Can be a slight help with some chores. Severe invalid.
- 10%—Totally dependent, helpless. Complete invalid.
  0%—Vegetative functions, such as swallowing, bladder and bowel functions, are not functioning. Bedridden.

Table 1.7 Unified Parkinsonism Rating Scale

NAME: _____

UNIT NUMBER: _____

DATES:	on/off	on/off	on/off	on/off	on/off	on/off	on/off	on/off
1. Mentation								
2. Thought disorder								
3. Depression								
4. Motivation/Initiative								
Subtotal #1-4								
5. Speech								
6. Salivation								
7. Swallowing								
8. Handwriting								
9. Cutting food								
10. Dressing								
11. Hygiene								
12. Turning in bed								
13. Falling								
14. Freezing								
15. Walking								

Table 1.7 Unified Parkinsonism Rating Scale (continued)

NAME: _____ UNIT NUMBER: _____

DATES:	on/off	on/off	on/off	on/off	on/off	on/off	on/off	on/off	on/off	on/off
16. Tremor										
17. Sensory symptoms										
Subtotal #5-17										
18. Speech										
19. Facial express.										
20. Tremor-at-rest										
face, lips, chin										
R/L hands										
R/L feet										
21. Action/Tremor R/L										
22. Rigidity										
neck										
R/L UE										
R/L LE										
23. Finger taps R/L										
24. Hand grips R/L										

Table 1.7 Unified Parkinsonism Rating Scale (continued)

NAME: _____ UNIT NUMBER: _____

DATES:	on/off	on/off	on/off	on/off	on/off	on/off	on/off	on/off	on/off
25. Hand pronation and supination R/L									
26. Leg agility R/L									
27. Arise from chair									
28. Posture									
29. Postural Stability									
30. Gait									
31. Body bradykinesia									
Subtotal #18-31									
Total Points: #1-31									
32. Dyskinesia—duration									
33. Dyskinesia—disability									
34. Dyskinesia—pain									
35. Early morning dystonia									
36. "Offs"—duration									
37. "Offs"—predict.									
38. "Offs"—unpredict.									

Table 1.7 Unified Parkinsonism Rating Scale (continued)

NAME: _____ UNIT NUMBER: _____

DATES:	on/off	on/off	on/off	on/off	on/off	on/off	on/off	on/off	on/off	on/off
39. "Offs"—sudden										
40. Anorexia, N, V										
41. Sleep disturbance										
42. Symptomatic orthostasis										
BP—sit/supine										
BP—standing										
Weight										
Pulse—sit/stand										
Hoehn & Yahr Stage										
% ADL Score (points)										
ADL (examiner's)										
Examiner's Initials										

REFERENCES

1. Adams RD, van Bogaert L, Vander Eecken H: Striato-nigral degeneration. J Neuropathol Exp Neurol 23:589-608, 1964.
2. Agnostoni E, Coletti A, Tredici O: Apraxia in deep cerebral lesions. J Neurol Neurosurg Psych 46:804-809, 1983.
3. Albert ML, Feldman RG, Willis AL: The subcortical dementia of progressive supranuclear palsy. J Neurol Neurosurg Psych 37:121- 130, 1974.
4. Appel SH: A unifying hypothesis for the cause of amyotrophic lateral sclerosis, parkinsonism and Alzheimer's disease. Ann Neurol 10:499-505, 1981.
5. Appenzeller O, Goss JE: Autonomic deficits in Parkinson's syndrome. Arch Neurol 24:50-57, 1971.
6. Barbeau A, Roy M: Familial subsets in idiopathic Parkinson's disease. Can J Neurol Sci 11:144-150, 1984.
7. Berenberg RA, Melen O, Howard GF, Hartner DH: Dominantly inherited ataxia with abnormal urinary glycolipid content. In Duvoisin RC, Plaitakis A. (Eds): The Olivopontocerebellar Atrophies. New York: Raven Press, pp 195-203, 1984.
8. Biemond A, Sinnege JLM: Tabes of Friedreich with degeneration of the substantia nigra, a special type of hereditary parkinsonism. Confinia Neurol 15:129-142, 1955.
9. Boller F, Passafiume D, Keefe N et al: Visuospatial impairment in Parkinson's disease. Role of perceptual and motor factors. Arch Neurol 41:485-490, 1984.
10. Brait K, Fahn S, Schwarz GA: Sporadic and familial parkinsonism and motor neuron disease. Neurology 23:990-1002, 1973.
11. Brown RG, Marsden DC: How common is dementia in Parkinson's disease? Lancet 2:1262-1265, 1984.
12. Burns RB, Chiueh CC, Markey SP, Ebert MH, Jacobowitz DM, KopinI J: A primate model of parkinsonism: selective destruction of dopaminergic neurons in the pars compacta of the substantia nigra by N-methyl-4-phenyl-1,2,3,6-tetrahydropyridine. Proc Natl Acad Sci USA 80:4546-4550, 1983.
13. Burns RS, Lewit PA, Ebert MH, Pakkenberg H, Kopin IJ: The clinical syndrome of striatal dopamine deficiency: parkinsonism induced by I-methyl-4-phenyl-1,2,3,6-tetrahydropyridine (MPTP). New Engl J Med 312:1418-1421, 1985.
14. Carlsson A, Lindquist M, Tagnusson T: 3,4-dihydroxy phenylalanine and 5-hydroxytryptophan as reserpine antagonists. Nature 180:1200, 1957.
15. Casson LR: Neurologic syndromes in boxers. NeuroView 1:1-4, 1985.
16. Cook DG, Fahn S, Brait KA: Chronic manganese intoxication. Arch Neurol 30:59-64, 1974.
17. Corsellis J, Burton C, Freeman-Browne D: The aftermath of boxing. Psychol Med 3:270-303, 1973.
18. Critchley M: Arteriosclerotic parkinsonism. Brain 52:23-83, 1929.
19. Davis GC, Williams AC, Markey SP, Ebert MH, Caine ED, Reichert CM, Kopin IJ: Chronic parkinsonism secondary to intravenous injection of meperidine analogues. Psychiatry Res 1:249-254, 1979.
20. Dejerine J, Thomas A: L'atrophie olivo-ponto-cerebelleuse. Nouv Iconogr Salpet 13:330-370, 1900.
21. Denny-Brown, D: The Basal Ganglia and Their Relation to Disorders of Movement. Oxford, Oxford University Press, 1962.

22. Ditter, SM, Mirra SS: Parkinson's disease features in Alzheimer's disease: a neuropathologic and clinical study. Neurology 36(suppl 1):225, 1986.

23. Drayer BP, Olanow W, Burger P, Johnson GA, Herfkens R, Riederer S: Parkinson plus syndrome: diagnosis using high field MR imaging of brain iron. Radiology 159:493-498, 1986.

24. Duvoisin RC: An apology and an introduction to the olivopontocerebellar atrophies. In Duvoisin RC, Plaitakis A (eds): The Olivopontocerebellar Atropies. New York: Raven Press, pp 5-12, 1984.

25. Fahr T: Idiopathische Verkalkung der Harngefasse. Centralbl f allg Path U Path Anat 50:129-133, 1930.

26. Gainotti G, Caltagirone C, Masullo C, Miceli G: Patterns of neuropsychologic impairment in various diagnostic groups of dementia. In Amaducci L, Davison AN, Antuono P (eds): Aging of the Brain and Dementia. New York: Raven Press, pp 245-250, 1980.

27. Goetz CG, Lutge W, Tanner C: Autonomic dysfunction in Parkinson's disease. Neurology 36:73-75, 1986.

28. Goetz CG, Tanner CM, Levy M, Wilson RS, Garron DG: Pain in idiopathic Parkinson's disease. Movement Disorders 1:45-50, 1986.

29. Gotham AM, Brown RG, Marsden CD: Depression in Parkinson's disease: a quantitative and qualitative analysis. J Neurol Neurosurg Psych 49(4):381-389, 1986.

30. Graham JG, Oppenheimer DR: Orthostatic hypotension and nicotine sensitivity in a case of multiple system atrophy. J Neurol Neurosurg Psy 32:28-34, 1969.

31. Grimes JD, Hassan MN, Preston DN: Adverse neurologic effects of metaclopramide. CMA Journ 126:23-52, 1982.

32. Hakim S, Adams RD: The special clinical problem of symptomatic hydrocephalus with normal cerebrospinal fluid pressure: observations on cerebrospinal fluid hemodyamics. J Neurol Sci 2:307-327, 1965.

33. Hallervorden J, Spatz H: Eigenartige erkrankung im extrapyramidalen system mit besonderer beiteiligung des globus pallidus und der substantia nigra. Z Neurol Psychiat 79:254-302, 1922.

34. Hoefer PF, Putnam TJ: Action potentials of muscles in rigidity and tremor. Arch Neurol Psych 43:704-725, 1940.

35. Hoehn MM, Yahr MD: Parkinsonism: onset, progression and mortality. Neurology 17:427-442, 1967.

36. Jankovic J, Kirkpatrick JB, Blomquist KA, Langlais PJ, Bird EP: Late-onset Hallervorden-Spatz Disease presenting as familial parkinsonism. Neurology 35:227-234, 1985.

37. Joachim CL, Morris J, Selkoe DJ: Autopsy neuropathology in 76 cases of clinically diagnosed Alzheimer's disease. Neurology 36(suppl 1):226, 1986.

38. Klawans HL: The Pharmacology of Extrapyramidal Movement Disorders. Basel, S. Karger, 1973.

39. Klawans HL, Stein RW, Tanner CM, Goetz CG: A pure parkinsonian syndrome following acute carbon monoxide poisoning. Arch Neurol 38:302-304, 1982.

40. Knutson E, Lying-Tunell V: Gait apraxia in normal-pressure hydrocephalus: patterns of movement and muscle activation. Neurology 35:155-160, 1985.

41. Koller WC: Sensory symptoms in Parkinson's disease. Neurology 34:957-959, 1984.

42. Konigsmark BW, Weiner LP: The olivopontocerebellar atrophies: a review. Medicine 49:227-241, 1970.
43. Kristensen MO: Progressive supranuclear palsy—20 years later. Acta Neurol Scand 71:177-189, 1985.
44. Kurlan R, Baker P, Miller C, Shoulson I: Severe compression neuropathy following sudden onset of parkinsonian immobility. Arch Neurol 42:720-721, 1985.
45. Langston JW, Ballard P, Tetrud JW, Irwin I: Chronic parkinsonism in humans due to a product of meperidine analog synthesis. Science 219:979-980, 1983.
46. Lepore FE, Duvoisin RC: "Apraxia" of eyelid opening: an involuntary levator inhibition. Neurology 35:423-427, 1985.
47. Leverenz J, Sumi M: Parkinson's disease in patients with Alzeheimer's disease. Arch Neurol 43:662-664, 1986.
48. Lewy FH: Neurological, medical and biochemical signs and symptoms indicating chronic industrial carbon disulphide absorption. Ann Int Med 15:869-883, 1941.
49. Marsden CD: The mysterious motor function of the basal ganglia. The Robert Wartenberg Lecture. Neurology 32:514-539, 1982.
50. Marsden CD: The pathophysiology of movement disorders. In Jancovic J (ed): Neurology Clinics, vol 2. Philadelphia: WB Saunders, pp 435-459, 1984.
51. Marsden CD: Defects of movement in Parkinson's disease. In Delwaide PJ, Agnoli A (eds): Clinical Neurophysiology in Parkinsonism. Amsterdam: Elsevier Science Publishers, pp 107-115, 1985.
52. Martland HS: Punch drunk: JAMA 91:1103-1107, 1928.
53. Mayeux R, Stern Y: Intellectual dysfunction and dementia in Parkinson's disease. In Mayeux R, Rosen WG (eds): The Dementias. New York: Raven Press, pp 211-227, 1983.
54. Mayeux R, Stern Y, Rosen J, Benson F: Is "subcortical dementia" a recognizable clinical entity? Ann Neurol 14:278-283, 1983.
55. McHugh PR, Folstein MF: Subcortical dementia. Address to the American Academy of Neurology, Boston, April, 1973.
56. Menzel P: Beitrag zur Kenntnis der hereditaren Ataxien und Kleinhirnatophie. Arch Psychiatr Nervenkr 22:160-190, 1891.
57. Moskowitz MA, Winickoff RN, Heinz EP: Familial calcifications of the basal ganglions. A metabolic and genetic study. New Eng J Med 185:72-77, 1971.
58. Narabayashi H, Nakamura R: Clinical neurophysiology of freezing in parkinsonism. In Delwaide PJ, Agnoli A (eds): Clinical Neurophysiology in parkinsonism. Amsterdam: Elsevier Science Publishers, pp 49-57, 1985.
59. Neill KG: An unusual case of syphilitic parkinsonism. Brit Med J 2:320-322, 1953.
60. Parkinson J: Essay on the Shaking Palsy. London: Sherwood, Neely and Jones, 1817.
61. Pastakia B, Polinsky R, DiChiro G, Simmons JT, Brown R, Weiner W: Multiple system atrophy (Shy-Drager Syndrome): MR imaging. Radiology 159:499-502, 1986.
62. Peters HA, Levine RL, Matthews CJ, Chapman LJ: Extrapyramidal symptoms from carbon disulphide exposure in grain storage workers. Neurology 36(suppl 1):342, 1981.
63. Peterson RC, Mokri B, Laws, ER: Surgical treatment of idiopathic hydrocephalus in elderly patients. Neurology 35:307-311, 1985.

64. Plaitakis A: Abnormal metabolism of neuroexcitatory amino acids in olivopontocerebellar atrophy. In Duvoisin RC, Plaitakis A (eds): The Olivopontocerebellar Atrophies. New York: Raven Press, pp 225-243, 1984.

65. Quinn NP, Perlmutter JS, Marsden CD: Acute administration of DL threoDOPS does not affect the freezing phenomenon in parkinsonian patients. Neurology 34(suppl):149, 1984.

66. Rajput AH, Offord KP, Beard CM, Durland LT: Epidemiology of parkinsonism: incidence, classification and mortality. Ann Neurol 16:278-282, 1984.

67. Rajput AH, Offord KP, Beard CM, Durland LT: A case-control study of smoking habits, dementia and other illnesses in idiopathic Parkinson's disease in Rochester, MN. Neurology 36(suppl 1):106, 1986.

68. Rebeiz JL, Kolodny EH, Richardson EP: Corticodentatonigral degeneration with neuronal achromasia. Arch Neurol 18:20-33, 1968.

69. Rodgers-Johnson P, Gerruot RM, Yanagihara R, Chen KM, Gajdusek DC, Gibbs CJ: Amyotrophic lateral sclerosis and parkinsonism-dementia on Guam: a 30 year evaluation of clinical and neuropathologic trends. Neurology 36:7-13, 1986.

70. Roos R, Gadjusek DC, Gibbs, CJ: The clinical characteristics of transmissable Creutzfeldt-Jakob disease. Brain 96:1-20, 1973.

71. Ropper AH: Case 23-1983, N Engl J Med 308:1406-1414, 1983.

72. Scheinberg IH, Sternlieb I: Wilson's Disease. Philadelphia: WB Saunders, pp 25-37, 1984.

73. Scheinberg IH, Sternlieb I: Wilson's Disease. Philadelphia: WB Saunders, pp 114-125, 1984.

74. Schwab RS, England AC: Projection technique for evaluating surgery in Parkinson's disease. In Gillingham FJ, Donaldson MC (eds): Third Symposium on Parkinson's Disease. Edinburgh: ES Livingston, pp 152-157, 1969.

75. Shy GM, Drager GA: A neurologic syndrome associated with orthostatic hypotension: a clinical-pathologic study. Arch Neurol 2:511-527, 1960.

76. Snider SR, Fahn S, Isgreen WP, Cote LJ: Primary sensory symptoms in parkinsonism. Neurology 26: 423-429, 1976.

77. Steele JC, Richardson JC, Olszewski J: Progressive supranuclear palsy: a heterogeneous degeneration involving the brainstem, basal ganglia and cerebellum with vertical gaze and pseduobulbar palsy, nuchal dystonia and dementia. Arch Neurol 10:333-359, 1964.

78. Stern M, Gur R, Saykin A, Hurtig H: The dementia of Parkinson's disease and Alzheimer's disease: is there a difference? J Am Ger Soc 34:475-478, 1986.

79. Sung JH, Mastri DR, Segal E: Pathology of Shy-Drager Syndrome. J Neuropathol Exp Neurol 38:353-368, 1979.

80. Swaiman KF, Smith SA, Trock GL, Siddiqui AR: Sea-blue histocytes, lymphocytic cytosomes, movement disorder, and 59 Fe-uptake in basal ganglia: Hallervorden-Spatz disease or ceroid storage disease with abnormal isotope scan. Neurology 33:301-305, 1983.

81. Takei Y, Mirra SS: Striatonigral degeneration: A form of multiple system atrophy with clinical parkinsonism. Prog Neuropath 2:217-251, 1973.

82. Taylor AE, Saint-Cyr JA, Lang AE, Kenney FT: Parkinson's disease and depression. A critical re-evaluation. Brain 109:279-292, 1986.

83. Todes DJ, Lees AJ: The pre-morbid personality of patients with Parkinson's disease. J Neur Neurosurg Psych 48:97-100, 1985.
84. Tolosa ES, Santamaria J: Parkinsonism and basal ganglia infarcts. Neurology 34:1516-1518, 1984.
85. Uitti RJ, Rajput AH, Ashenburst EM, Rozdilsky B: Cyanide-induced parkinsonism: A clinicopathologic report. Neurology 35:921-925, 1985.
86. van Eck, JH: Parkinsonism as a misleading brain tumor syndrome. Psychiat Neurol Neurochir 64:109-123, 1961.
87. Victor M, Adams RD, Cole M: The acquired (non-Wilsonian) type of chronic hepatocerebral degeneration. Medicine 44:345-396, 1965.
88. Von Economo C: Encephalitis lethargica. New York: Oxford University Press, 1931.
89. Wilson SAK: Progressive lenticular degeneration: a familial nervous disease associated with cirrhosis of the liver. Brain 34:295-507, 1912.
90. Zetusky WJ, Jancovic J, Pirozzolo FJ: The heterogeneity of Parkinson's disease: clinical and prognostic implications. Neurology 35:522-526, 1985.
91. Ziegler DIS, Schimke RN, Kepes JJ, Rose DL, Klinkerfuss G: Late onset ataxia, rigidity and peripheral neuropathy. A familial syndrome with variable therapeutic response to levodopa. Arch Neurol 27:52-66, 1972.

Chapter 2

The Epidemiology and Natural History of Parkinson's Disease

Lawrence I. Golbe and Roger C. Duvoisin

INTRODUCTION

A COMPREHENSIVE CONSIDERATION OF THE practical management of Parkinson's disease should include a discussion of its epidemiology and natural history. The present debate over when to begin treatment with dopaminergics, to cite one example, pivots on an understanding of the course of the native disease. The introduction of levodopa in the early 1970s has obscured the natural history of the disease from younger neurologists, who in most cases prescribe levodopa without benefit of personal experience of the course of the underlying morbid process.

The hope of Parkinson's disease (PD) prophylaxis (or amelioration) offered by study of MPTP and other potential exogenous causative agents relies on epidemiological investigation of premorbid toxic exposure, even if constitutional factors also play a role.

The epidemiological question that has confronted every neurologist in the consulting room concerns the heritability of PD. Genetic studies of PD hold not only prognostic value to relatives, but also will be important in identification of at-risk persons who might benefit from future efforts at disease prophylaxis.

PREVALENCE

Until the 1960s little was known of the epidemiology of PD apart from postencephalitic parkinsonism. The cohort theory of Poskanzer and Schwab [45] held that most cases of PD were sequelae of the encephalitis pandemic following World War I and that the disease would disappear with the passing of that generation. Periodic surveys of the Rochester, Minnesota population since 1935 [30,47] have shown no decrease in disease prevalence (all cases) or incidence (new cases) nor any change in the age distribution of the disease over time. The annual age- and sex-adjusted incidence of new cases in Rochester has remained stable at approximately 20 per 100,000 population for the past 50 years. These observations are incompatible with the post-encephalitic cohort theory, which has now been laid to rest.

The prevalence of PD in surveys among Western populations has ranged from 65 to 187 per 100,000 population [4,5,14,23,29,38,44]. The highest figures are from Rochester and from Iceland, where more complete ascertainment might be permitted by an efficient, linked medical records system. However, a more recent door-to-door survey of the entire population of a rural county in Mississippi by Schoenberg et al. [53] found a prevalence of 130 per 100,000 inhabitants. That study found the prevalence of "possible" or "definite" idiopathic PD in the population over age 40 to be 200 per 100,000. Comparison across studies is hampered by differences in methods of case ascertainment, diagnostic criteria, population age distributions, availability of chronic care for debilitated patients (producing differential postdiagnosis survival which affects prevalence, but not incidence), inclusion of multiple system atrophies, postencephalitic and "arteriosclerotic" parkinsonism, and varying use of phenothiazines.

Differences in PD prevalence across ethnic lines are a matter of some disagreement. Studies in Africa [35,48] and Baltimore [26] found rates among blacks to be significantly lower than among whites, though serious questions of completeness of case ascertainment arise for these studies. A study of PD in Sardinians [50], who share some ancestry and HLA antigens with Africans, show a PD risk intermediate between those of white and black populations. Complicating (or perhaps simplifying) the picture is the Mississippi study [53], which found no racial difference in age-adjusted prevalence. The latter authors surmise that all the other studies' reliance on medical records and physicians' reports rather than door-to-door survey accounts for the discrepant findings among groups with differing access to medical care. It is likely that the observation of higher PD mortality in the northern and western U.S. than in the southern and eastern areas [30] is secondary to differences in case ascertainment along racial lines.

A survey of medical records in a medium-size Japanese city [17] validated by a door-to-door survey of one district found the age-adjusted prevalence rate to be 81 per 100,000. An even lower rate was found in a door-to-door survey of 63,000 subjects in 6 urban centers in the People's Republic of China, 57 per 100,000 after age adjustment [33]. The next logical step would seem to be a door-to- door study of an American population of Oriental origin. Though neuromelanin is not identical with cutaneous melanin, the dissociation of degree of skin pigmentation from degeneration of a pigmented neural structure is an interesting and important issue.

The resurgence of interest in a toxic etiology following the description of MPTP-induced parkinsonism has led epidemiologists to seek out small geographic or demographic foci of increased PD prevalence. Recent evidence [46] suggests that PD is more common in rural than urban areas (see below).

The notion of a toxic etiology attaches new importance to accurate measurement of PD incidence: Such surveys, repeated over time, may permit correlation with the introduction into that area of new industrial or agricultural toxins. It is interesting that despite its (modern) frequency and striking clinical appearance, PD was not described until the early Industrial Revolution. All of Shakespeare's alleged references to parkinsonism seem, on our reading, to be more compatible with essential or senile tremor.

NATURAL HISTORY

Though the natural history of idiopathic PD probably has not changed since the time of Parkinson himself, published surveys of the age distribution since the 1920s have been biased toward younger patients. Admixture of large numbers of (usually young) postencephalitics, lesser availability of medical care to the elderly, and a tendency to refer younger patients to academic centers have together been responsible for this artifact. With lessening influence of at least the first two factors, the mean age at diagnosis is now 60 to 65, with onset of symptoms some 5 years before. Approximately 2% of patients with PD are diagnosed before age 50.

The introduction of levodopa has profoundly influenced the subsequent clinical course of PD. This was documented by Hoehn, who tabulated disease progression both before [19] and after [20] widespread use of levodopa using similar methods of analysis. She found that the patients spent 3 to 5 years longer at each Hoehn-Yahr stage than before levodopa, though the proportion of patients at each stage was unchanged by treatment. The average age at death increased from 66 to 72. Most importantly, whereas 60% of patients before levodopa became disabled (Stage IV or V) or died between 5 and 10 years after diagnosis, after levodopa this figure declined to 25%.

This study must be interpreted carefully, however. Because the postlevodopa group includes only those patients actually treated with the drug, it may be biased against patients with dementia or other concurrent illness that may have contraindicated levodopa while leading to earlier disability or death. A community-based survey of patients treated with levodopa [47] partially avoids this pitfall by comparing postdiagnosis annual mortality rates of treated patients with non-PD age-matched community controls. Mortality for the two groups did not differ significantly. Although this is an important finding, the authors point out that neither it nor any other study has proven that levodopa has prolonged life expectancy among parkinsonians.

The opposite question is of central importance in guiding management of PD: Does levodopa accelerate the long-term clinical course of the disease? Markham and Diamond [37] found that parkinsonian disability progresses in approximately linear fashion for at least 14 years after symptom onset and that the rate of progression is the same regardless of the interval between the onset of symptoms and the start of levodopa therapy. Their subjects, whether treated or untreated, progressed approximately 4% of the total span of their disability scale per year. Institution of levodopa at any point in the disease progression produced an improvement equivalent to 25-30% of the total span of the scale. Expressed differently, levodopa improved neurologic function in every patient, regardless of the point in the progression of the disease at which levodopa was introduced. The authors interpret their findings as support for early use of levodopa in PD. They did not report their patients' progress beyond the halfway point in their disability scale, so could not comment on the effect of levodopa on the incidence of severe disability or death.

Our interpretation of the available mortality data is that levodopa-responsive PD patients experience mortality similar to that of the non-PD population for 8 to 10 years after initiation of treatment. Thereafter the mortality ratio rises to approximately 2:1.

GENETIC STUDIES

Concurrent with such descriptive epidemiological studies of PD, analytical epidemiological studies have proceeded apace in a search for the cause of the disease. The diminished appeal of a genetic component and a new suspicion of an environmental agent are the two arms of the recent revolution in the analytical epidemiology of PD.

Surveys since the turn of the century have found the frequency of a positive family history among parkinsonians to range from 15% to 20% [7]. However, these studies have suffered from failure to control for the number of relatives considered in the history and from failure to exclude families with essential tremor and OPCA. Mjones' influential study [40], in particular, suffered from inclusion of many oligosymptomatic (or "incipient") secondary cases, even when the illness in those individuals began years earlier than in the proband. When such doubtful secondary cases are excluded, the percentage of affected siblings in Mjones' series falls from 7.2% to 3.1% [9].

Recalculation of the frequency of PD among siblings in Mjones' study now yields a figure very close to the 2.5% lifetime incidence of parkinsonism observed by Kurland [29] in his landmark study of the prevalence of parkinsonism in the Rochester, Minnesota population. One of us (RCD) reviewed the family histories of 207 personal patients with typical PD and found the frequency of PD in patients' parents, almost all of whom were deceased, to be 3.6%, a figure not very different from Kurland's population-based study. In fact, when a correction is made for the ascertainment bias whereby an ill individual is more likely to have carefully scrutinized his family history, the difference becomes even less.

However, such retrospective surveys are weakened by an inability to examine personally all of the at-risk relatives to avoid false-negative reports in individuals whose parkinsonism, by virtue of poor access to medical care, may have been interpreted as normal senile changes or cerebrovascular disease. Duvoisin et al. [8] personally examined siblings of patients and siblings of their spouses in a standardized manner. Parkinsonism was found in 4 of 146 patient siblings and in 3 of 145 spouse siblings, suggesting that there is no significant heritable component in the etiology of PD. Even the pedigrees of "familial Parkinson's disease" reported by Roy et al. [51] reveal a lifetime incidence of PD among first-degree relatives of only 2.9%. (The authors considered essential tremor in relatives as evidence for the existence of the "essential tremor-related parkinsonism" discussed above.)

Convincing as family studies may be, PD is sufficiently rare that a slight genetic contribution can be missed if the number of at-risk relatives surveyed is too small. Probands' parents are usually deceased and their children are usually too young to be at significant risk for displaying clinical signs. Therefore, siblings comprise the only first-degree relatives available for careful survey. A family study would therefore have to be prohibitively large to avoid Type II error in uncovering a modest genetic factor. A twin study is a much more powerful technique for a disease of the prevalence of PD.

Ward et al. [55] reported a series of 43 patients with PD who were members of genotypically confirmed monozygotic twin pairs. Only 2 of the pairs were found, on careful standardized personal examination, to be concordant for PD, and one of these pairs had atypical PD. The maximum concordance rate was therefore only 4.7%, which excludes a significant genetic factor in PD pathogenesis. The reader of subsequent isolated reports [22,27] of monozygotic twins concordant for PD must ask whether such pairs are outnumbered 30- or 40-fold by unreported discordant twin pairs.

MPTP, SMOKING AND PERSONALITY

At the same time as a significant genetic component in the cause of PD was becoming less likely, a relatively simple pyridine derivative, 1-methyl-4-phenyl-1,2,3,6-tetrahydropyridine (MPTP), a by-product of synthetic-heroin synthesis, was serendipitously observed to cause a disease very similar to PD [6,31]. The widespread environmental distribution of natural and synthetic pyridines raises the intriguing possibility that an MPTP analogue may be the cause of PD. Even more intriguing is the hope that an MPTP analogue may be found that would competitively inhibit the toxin's neural uptake mechanism.

A negative association of PD and cigarette smoking has been known since the 1960s [16,24]. Cigarette smoke contains dozens of pyridine analogues, including 4-phenyl-pyridine [18], which closely resembles methyl-phenyl-pyridinium, the toxic metabolite of MPTP [36]. If the smoking-PD dissociation is both genuine and causative, a possibility for PD treatment or prophylaxis exists.

That the smoking-PD dissociation was not merely an artifact of differential mortality among smokers (who might tend to die before an age where PD is likely to occur) was established in five separate case-control studies [3,12,25,39,41]. One of these [41], a cooperative Veterans Administration study, was criticized as merely demonstrating an unusually high prevalence of smoking in the control population; another [3] was reanalyzed by its authors [15] and found to reveal no difference in cumulative nicotine intake between patients and controls. However, all five studies found that the likelihood of a PD patient having smoked cigarettes before symptom onset to be significantly less than that of controls at an equivalent age. The twin study [55] mentioned above also found that probands were less likely to have smoked than their unaffected cotwins, and if both smoked, the proband usually smoked less. Both findings were statistically significant. The smoking-PD dissociation was disputed by the findings of Rajput [47], but 14.5% of his patient group had parkinsonisms other than PD. The 7.2% with drug-induced parkinsonism, in particular, may have had an unusually high prevalence of smoking often found in schizophrenia and other psychiatric illness, thereby raising the smoking rate among the parkinsonians to "normal."

Experimental evidence for an anti-PD effect of cigarette smoke is that nicotine increases dopamine turnover in rat striatum [11] and increases firing rates of rat nigral neurons [34].

Although one of us (RCD), in unpublished observations found that nicotine did not help PD symptoms at least over the short term in a series of two patients, other workers have found cigarette smoking or nicotine chewing gum to produce "remarkable" but transient improvement of symptoms in 5 juvenile parkinsonians in an open trial [21].

To test the hypothesis that the smoking-PD dissociation is causative, we surveyed a large number of parkinsonians in search of a dose-response relationship between increasing intensity of smoking (during the premorbid years) and decreasing severity of subsequent parkinsonism [13]. Using several measures of smoking intensity and amount, we found no correlation with rate of PD-symptom progression, age at symptom onset, or nature of the predominant symptom, and concluded that the smoking-PD dissociation is probably not causal in origin.

The most likely explanation for this inverse association, in the opinion of most workers, is personality. Retrospective assessments of personality in parkinsonians [42,43] and the twin study [55] found that the patients were more likely than controls (or cotwins) to have a morally conservative, rule-abiding, passive, and dour personality, even since adolescence. Because nonsmokers' personality traits [52] often overlap those of parkinsonians, it seems likely that a presymptomatic stage of PD includes such personality traits, which in turn tend to cause nonsmoking. Against this interpretation is Kondo's recent case-control study of premorbid risk factors [28] that found, on multivariate analysis, that nonsmoking and rigid personality were independent risk factors.

ENVIRONMENTAL RISK FACTORS

One possible conclusion from the personality data is admittedly indirect but of pivotal importance: The agent causing PD acts at least as early as preadolescence, when the personality is solidified. An alternative conclusion is that persons of a "preparkinsonian" personality may become exposed to a PD-causing agent (or fail to expose themselves to a protective agent) later in life. Though the twin study failed to detect differential environmental exposures early in life, anamnestic data from many decades past may not be reliable. One possible solution is a series of PD-discordant juvenile-onset PD twin pairs, who might have better access to data on childhood environmental exposure.

A more practical but less elegant solution would be a case-control study of kindreds with many juvenile-onset parkinsonians. Rajput's [46] case-control study of risk factors in juvenile-onset (though nonfamilial) PD found a significantly greater likelihood in the PD subjects of having been raised in a rural area rather than in a town. (The survey was performed in Saskatchewan, Canada, where there are no large cities.) The authors mention well-water use as one environmental factor that occurred consistently in the rural but not the "urban" group.

Other workers have sought early-life environmental risk factors. Recent labor-atory studies show increased susceptibility to DNA breakage by ionizing radiation in cultured neuronal lines from brains of patients with PD. Nevertheless, when Kondo [28] measured PD incidence among atom-bomb survivors from Hiroshima and Nagasaki, no relation of PD risk to radiation dose emerged. Longer-term follow-up of these cohorts is in progress.

Tanner [54], inspired by the positive findings in Saskatchewan, surveyed a large group of parkinsonians and found that patients with onset by age 47 were significantly more likely to have lived in a rural area and to have used well water. Barbeau et al. [2] identified geographic foci in Quebec of PD prevalence as much as four times that in the lowest-prevalence areas of the province. The high-prevalence areas were those where market-gardening and pulp and paper mills are located. These activities employ pesticides and/or fungicides, which, the authors surmised, may be the thread that binds the observations of rural living and well-water use. They found the correlation between incidence of PD and pesticide use to be .967 (cited by Lewin [32]). In support of this hypothesis, these authors have found a deficiency in a certain hepatic detoxification process in many PD patients. Though these observations are as yet unconfirmed, they may point the way to the ultimate maneuver in PD management: prevention through removal of a man-made environmental toxin. Enthusiasm for this line of investigation must be tempered by the observations of the twin study [55] where all twins lived together at least until the age of 19. For an exogenous toxin to begin acting on the individual after that age seems, in light of the personality studies and existence of juvenile PD, to be unlikely. Eldridge [10] attempts to resolve this paradox. Citing the asymmetric occurrence of some congenital defects in monozygotic twins, he proposes the novel hypothesis that monozygotic twins may receive unequal amounts of a "protective factor" in utero that may confer differential susceptibility to an exogenous toxin acting during childhood.

Epidemiological study of a disease ordinarily associated with the senium has now led us back to the womb. Nongenetic gestational factors are poorly understood, but have been addressed by neuroepidemiologists studying epilepsy, cerebral palsy, the rubella syndrome, and neural tube defects. Improvements in prenatal care have provided some measure of prophylaxis against these disorders. However, the long postnatal latency of PD may render intrauterine etiological factors, even if they exist, undetectable.

The issue of the interaction of PD and pregnancy, therefore, like many aspects of the analytical epidemiology of PD, is a field where much is still speculative, but where issues fundamental to the etiology and hope for prevention of PD may lie.

REFERENCES

1. Barbeau A, Roy MN, Paris S, Cloutier T, Plasse L, Poirier J: Ecogenetics of Parkinson's disease: 4-hydroxylation of debrisoquine. Lancet 2:1213-16, 1985.
2. Barbeau A, Roy M: Genetic susceptibility, environmental factors and Parkinson's disease. VIIIth International Symposium on Parkinson's Disease, 1985, p 13.
3. Baumann RJ, Jameson, HD, McKean HE, Haack DG, Weisberg LM: Cigarette smoking and Parkinson's disease: 1. A comparison of cases with matched neighbors. Neurology 30:839-43, 1980.
4. Brewis M, Poskanzer DC, Rolland C, et al: Neurological disease in an English city. Acta Neurol Scand 42(Suppl 24):1-89, 1966.
5. Broman T: Parkinson's syndrome: prevalence and incidence in Goteborg. Acta Neurol Scand 39(Suppl 4):95-101, 1963.
6. Davis GC, Williams AC, Markey SP, Ebert MH, Caine ED, Reichert CM, Kopin IJ: Chronic parkinsonism secondary to intravenous injection of meperidine analogues. Psychiatry Res 1:249-254, 1979.
7. Duvoisin RC, Yahr MD, Schweitzer MD, Merritt HH: Parkinsonism before and since the epidemic of encephalitis lethargica. Arch Neurol 9:232, 1963.

8. Duvoisin RC, Gearing FR, Schweitzer MD, Yahr MD: A family study of parkinsonism. In Barbeau A, Brunette JR (eds): Progress in Neurogenetics. Excerpta Medica (Amsterdam), pp 492-496, 1969.
9. Duvoisin RC. Is Parkinson's disease acquired or inherited? Can J Neurol Sci 11(Suppl):151-155, 1984.
10. Eldridge R, Ince S: The low concordance rate for Parkinson's disease in twins: a possible explanation. Neurology 34:1354-1356, 1984.
11. Giorguieff-Chesselet MR, Kemel ML, Wandscheer D, Glowinski J: Regulation of dopamine release by presynaptic nicotinic receptors in rat striatal slices: effect of nicotine in a low concentration. Life Sci 25:1267-1262, 1979.
12. Godwin-Austen RB, Lee PN, Marmot MG, Stern GM: Smoking and Parkinson's disease. J Neurol Neurosurg Psych 45:577-581, 1982.
13. Golbe LI, Cody RA, Duvoisin RC: Smoking and Parkinson's disease: search for a dose-response relationship. Arch Neurol 43:774-778, 1986.
14. Gudmundsson KRA: A clinical survey of parkinsonism in Iceland. Acta Neurol Scand 43(Suppl 33):9-61, 1967.
15. Haack DG, Baumann RJ, McKean HE, et al: Nicotine exposure and Parkinson's disease. Am J Epidemiol 114:191-200, 1981.
16. Hammond CA: Smoking in relation to the death rates of one million men and women. In Epidemiologic Approaches to the Study of Cancer and Other Chronic Disease. Monograph No. 19, Natl Cancer Inst. Washington, DC: U.S. Govt Printing Office, p 127-204, 1966.
17. Harada H, Nishikawa S, Takahashi K: Epidemiology of Parkinson's disease in a Japanese city. Arch Neurol 40:151-154, 1983.
18. Heckman R, Best F: An investigation of lipophilic bases of cigarette smoke condensate. Tobacco Sci 125:33-39, 1981.
19. Hoehn MM, Yahr MD: Parkinsonism: onset, progression, and mortality. Neurology 17:427-42, 1967.
20. Hoehn MM: Result of chronic levodopa therapy and its modification by bromocriptine in Parkinson's disease. Acta Neurol Scand 71:97- 106, 1985.
21. Ishikawa A, Miyatake T: Smoking efficacy in five cases of juvenile parkinsonism. VIIIth International Symposium on Parkinson's Disease, 1985, p 98.
22. Jankovic J, Reches A: Parkinson's disease in monozygotic twins. Ann Neurol 19:405-408, 1986.
23. Jenkins AC: Epidemiology of parkinsonism in Victoria. Med J Aust 2:496-502, 1966.
24. Kahn HA: The Dorn study of smoking and mortality among U.S. veterans. In Epidemiologic Approaches to the Study of Cancer and Other Chronic Disease. Monograph No. 19, Natl Cancer Inst. Washington, DC: U.S. Govt Printing Office, pp 1-125, 1966.
25. Kessler II, Diamond EL: Epidemiologic studies of Parkinson's disease. I. Smoking and Parkinson's disease: a survey and explanatory hypothesis. Am J Epidemiol 94:16-25, 1971.
26. Kessler II: Epidemiological study of Parkinson's disease: III. A community-based survey. Am J Epidemiol 96:242-254, 1972.
27. Koller W, O'Hara R, Nutt J, Young J, Rubino F: Monozygotic twins with Parkinson's disease. Ann Neurol 19:402-404, 1986.

28. Kondo K: Epidemiological evaluation of the risk factors to Parkinson's disease. VIIIth International Symposium on Parkinson's Disease, 1985, p 48.

29. Kurland LT: Descriptive epidemiology of selected neurologic and myopathic disorders with particular reference to a survey in Rochester, Minnesota. J Chron Dis 8:378-418, 1958.

30. Kurland LT, Kurtzke JF, Goldberg ID: Epidemiology of Neurologic and Sense Organ Disorders (Chap 3, Parkinsonism). Cambridge, MA, Harvard University Press, 1973.

31. Langston JW, Ballard P, Tetrud JW, Irwin I: Chronic parkinsonism in humans due to a product of meperidine-analog synthesis. Science 219:979-980, 1983.

32. Lewin R: Parkinson's disease: an environmental cause? Science 229:257-258, 1985.

33. Li S, Schoenberg BS, Wang C, Cheng X, Rui D, Bolis CL, Schoenberg DG: A prevalence survey of Parkinson's disease and other movement disorders in the People's Republic of China. Arch Neurol 42:655-657, 1985.

34. Lichtensteiger W, Hefti F, Felix D, Huwyler T, Melamed E, Schlumpf M: Stimulation of nigrostriatal dopamine neurones by nicotine. Neuropharmacology 21:963-968, 1982.

35. Lombard A, Gelfand M: Parkinson's disease in the African. Centr Afr J Med 24:5-8, 1978.

36. Markey SP, Johannessen JN, Chiueh CC, et al: Intraneuronal generation of a pyridinium metabolite may cause drug-induced parkinsonism. Nature 311:464-467, 1984.

37. Markham C, Diamond S: Evidence to support early levodopa therapy in Parkinson's disease. Neurology 31:125-131, 1981.

38. Marttila RJ, Rinne UK: Epidemiology of Parkinson's disease in Finland. Acta Neurol Scand 53:81-102, 1976.

39. Marttila RJ, Rinne UK: Smoking and Parkinson's disease. Acta Neurol Scand 62:322-325, 1980.

40. Mjones H: Paralysis agitans: a clinical genetic study. Acta Psychiat et Neurol Scand 25(Suppl 54):1-195, 1949.

41. Nefzger MD, Quadfasel FA, Karl VC: A retrospective study of smoking in Parkinson's disease. Am J Epidemiol 88:149-158, 1968.

42. Ogawa T: Personality characteristics of Parkinson's disease. Percep Motor Skills 52:375-378, 1981.

43. Poewe W, Gerstenbrand F, Ransmayr G, Plorer S: Premorbid personality of Parkinson patients. J Neural Transm, (Suppl 19):215-242, 1983.

44. Pollock M, Hornabrook RW: The prevalence, natural history and dementia of Parkinson's disease. Brain 89:429-448, 1966.

45. Poskanzer DC, Schwab RW: Cohort analysis of Parkinson's syndrome: evidence for a single etiology related to subclinical infection about 1920. J Chron Dis 16:961-973, 1963.

46. Rajput AH, Stern W, Christ A, Laverty W: Etiology of Parkinson's disease: environmental factor(s). Neurology 34(Suppl 1):207, 1984.

47. Rajput AH, Offord KP, Beard CM, Kurland LT: Epidemiology of parkinsonism: incidence, classification, and mortality. Ann Neurol 16:278-282, 1984.

48. Reef HE: Prevalence of Parkinson's disease in a multiracial community. In Jager HWA, Bruyn GW, Heijhstee AP (eds): 11th World Congress of Neurology, Excerpta Medica (Amsterdam) 1977, p 125.
49. Robbins JH, Otsuka F, Tarone RE, Polinsky RJ, Brumback RA, Nee LA: Parkinson's disease and Alzheimer's disease: hypersensitivity to x-rays in cultured cell lines. J Neurol Neurosurg Psychiatry 48:916-923, 1985.
50. Rosati G, Graniere E, Pinna L, Aiello I, Tola R, De Bastiani P, Pirisi A, Devoto MC: The risk of Parkinson's disease in Mediterranean people. Neurology 30:250-255, 1980.
51. Roy M, Boyer L, Barbeau A: A prospective study of 50 cases of familial Parkinson's disease. Can J Neurol Sci 10:37-42, 1983.
52. Royal College of Physicians. Smoking or Health. London, Pitman Medical, 1977.
53. Schoenberg BS, Anderson DW, Haerer AF: Prevalence of Parkinson's disease in the biracial population of Copiah County, Mississippi, Neurology 35:841-845, 1985.
54. Tanner CM: Influence of environmental factors on the onset of Parkinson's disease. Neurology 36(Suppl 1):215, 1986.
55. Ward CD, Duvoisin RC, Ince SE, Nutt JD, Eldridge R, Calne DB: Parkinson's disease in 65 pairs of twins and in a set of quadruplets. Neurology 33:815-824, 1983.

Chapter 3

Biochemical Pathology and Pharmacology of Parkinson's Disease

James P. Bennett

OUR UNDERSTANDING OF THE NEUROCHEMICAL abnormalities present in patients with neurodegenerative disease, including idiopathic Parkinson's disease (PD), has increased concomitantly with our knowledge of chemical substances used in synaptic transmission. The first group of substances characterized as neurotransmitters in mammalian brain were the biogenic amines: norepinephrine (NE), dopamine (DA), and serotonin (5-hydroxytryptamine, 5-HT). The hypothesis that these chemicals might be utilized by central nervous system synapses derived from extensive evidence of their utilization as transmitters in the peripheral (autonomic) nervous system and gastrointestinal tract. The development of sensitive, simple fluorometric assays for DA, NE, and 5-HT enabled the measurement of regional levels of these substances in brain. Investigators found that these chemicals were widely distributed throughout the forebrain, with each substance having a unique regional distribution. During the same period, Swedish anatomists at the Karolinska Institute in Stockholm found that DA, NE, and 5-HT in freeze-dried brain tissue exposed to hot formaldehyde vapor fluoresced at unique excitation wavelengths and could be localized anatomically.

During the middle and late 1960s results of neurochemical analyses and histofluorescent anatomical studies merged to produce a consistent pattern of organization of mammalian biogenic amine neurotranmitter systems. The neuronal cell bodies of origin for the entire forebrain contents of DA, NE, and 5-HT were found to be located in the brainstem in discrete nuclear groups. Axon bundles containing each amine ascended rostrally, giving off nerve endings to forebrain subcortical structures (i.e., thalamus, hypothalamus, striatum, globus pallidus) and diffuse terminal innervation to the cerebral cortical mantle.

At this time, an important principle of aminergic innervation was appreciated; small compact brainstem nuclei exerted extensive "control" over the forebrain. Physiological studies of these aminergic nuclei provided further support for this theme. Recordings of firing patterns of individual neurons manufacturing DA (in the substantia nigra of the ventral midbrain), 5-HT (in the dorsal and medial raphe nuclei of the midline midbrain), and NE (in the locus ceruleus under the floor of the fourth ventricle) consistently showed slow, regular 4-8 Hz firing rates [7]. Such data suggested that the forebrain is constantly influenced by the tonic release of DA, NE, and 5-HT neurotranmitters. This mode of neuronal firing and neurotranmitter action is quite different from the rapid on-off excitatory and inhibitory events that characterize the majority of synaptic transmissions in the forebrain.

Postmortem studies suggest that all three aminergic neurotransmitter systems (DA, NE, and 5-HT) are directly or indirectly affected by the degenerative pathology of PD. Variations occur in the degree and consistency of involvmeent, with DA loss being the greatest and most consistent (indeed, a sine qua non of PD). As will be discussed, other major neurotranmitters systems are affected in PD. For some of these systems, (for instance, gamma-aminobutyric acid (GABA)), decreased function appears to be of pathophysiological significance. For other chemical systems, alterations in PD brains are of unclear significance.

PARKINSON'S DISEASE, DOPAMINE METABOLISM, AND RATIONAL DOPAMINE REPLACEMENT

The mammalian basal ganglia are composed of several large subcortical forebrain nuclei including the caudate and putamen (collectively referred to as corpus striatum), globus pallidus, subthalamic nucleus, certain anterior and ventral thalamic "motor" nuclei, and the substantia nigra in the ventral midbrain. The idea that PD might be associated with dysfunction of the basal ganglia can be traced to the clinicopathological correlations of Kinnier Wilson [35] and the early neuropathological descriptions of pigmented-nerve cell loss in the zona compacta of the substantia nigra [14]. Pioneering chemical analyses of postmortem PD brains by Hornekiewicz et al. suggested that the symptoms of PD arose as a result of forebrain DA deficiency [15,16]. Patients who died in the earliest stages

Table 3.1 Neurochemistry of Parkinson's Disease: Regional Dopamine (DA),
Homovanillic Acid (HVA) Levels and Tyrosine Hydroxylase (TH) and DOPA
Decarboxylase (DDC) Activities in Postmortem Brains*

Brain region	Control Values (%)				
	DA	HVA	HVA/DA	TH	DDC
Putamen	2.8	11	400	18	7.5
Caudate	4.9	41	780	17	15
Substantia nigra	15.0	18	120	35	3.9

*Data derived from reference 16.

of PD had already lost about 75-80% of the zona compacta neurons and
DA content in the nigra and striatum [5]. Patients who died with far-advanced PD had few if any remaining zona compacta neurons and little detectable striatal DA.

The concept that PD is a clinical syndrome totally explainable by striatal DA deficiency has recently received additional support from a tragic experiment by both man and nature. Several dozen heroin addicts, primarily in California, have accidentally been exposed over the last 4 to 5 years to N-methyl, 4-phenyl tetrahydropyridine (MPTP), a by-product in the synthesis of a meperidine analogue. Several of these individuals have developed severe clinical parkinsonism, indistinguishable from idiopathic PD [1,8]. This syndrome of MPTP-induced parkinsonism has been reported in primates. Postmortem histological analysis of these primates' brains [18] and of the one known human case [11] have shown marked loss of substantia nigra dopaminergic neurons and no other consistent alterations. Chemical studies demonstrated profound DA depletion in nigra, caudate, and putamen of a magnitude similar to that found in patients dying with severe idiopathic PD (see Tables 3.1 and 3.2). In the chronic phase of MPTP-induced parkinsonism, DA levels remain re-

Table 3.2 Effects of MPTP Treatment on Monkey Caudate
Dopamine Levels*

Severity of parkinsonism	Control DA levels (%)
None (control)	100
Subclinical	50
Moderate	24
Severe	3

*Date derived from reference 8.

duced, whereas levels of other biogenic amines and their metabolites tend
to return toward control values [9]. Thus, the MPTP model has provided
unequivocal evidence that all of the motor deficits of idiopathic PD can
arise solely from depletion of striatal DA.

Dopamine is synthesized from the dietary amino acid L-tyrosine first
by hydroxylation of the tyrosine ring (See Figure 3.1). This reaction uses
molecular oxygen, is catalyzed by the enzyme tyrosine hydroxylase (TO-
Hase), and leads to the formation of L-3,4 dihydroxyphenylalanine
(levodopa). Under normal circumstances, the hydroxylation of tyrosine is
the rate-limiting step in DA synthesis, and TH enzyme is found only in
neurons and nerve endings that manufacture DA or NE. Once formed,
levodopa is rapidly decarboxylated to dopamine by dopa decarboxylase
enzyme (DDC), which will decarboxylate a variety of aromatic amino
acids. DDC is found in biogenic amine neurons and terminals, and also in
some striatal neurons that do not appear to manufacture biogenic amines
[21]. In NE neurons and endings, DA is subsequently hydroxylated in the
beta position of the alkyl chain by dopamine beta-hydroxylase (DBH) to
yield NE. In the brain DBH is localized to neuronal populations that manufacture NE.

Once synthesized, DA can be stored in small vesicles that actively transport DA into them. These vesicles are generally located in the presynaptic nerve endings of dopaminergic neurons and are sensitive to drugs, such
as reserpine and tetrabenazine, that cause depletion of vesicular DA
stores. Current evidence supports the hypothesis that vesicular DA is primarily a storage form of the neurotransmitter and is not actively involved
in normal minute-to-minute synaptic transmission. Newly synthesized DA
appears to be preferentially released under physiological circumstances
whereas vesicular DA stores can be mobilized at times of physiological or
pharmacological stress.

DA is normally synthesized exclusively in intraneuronal compartments,
but its catabolism involves a variety of neuronal and nonneuronal
processes (see Figure 3.1). Oxidative deamination of DA by monoamine
oxidase enzyme (MAO) is believed to take place primarily in neuronal
compartments and yields dihydroxyphenlacetic acid (DOPAC). Once released outside the neuron or nerve ending, DA can be catabolized by cate-
chol-O-methyltransferase (COMT) to 3-methoxytyramine (30MT). Both
MAO and COMT activities are found in brain and in many other non-
nervous tissues, particularly liver. There is significant COMT activity in
red blood cells as well. Once formed, DOPAC is a substrate for COMT

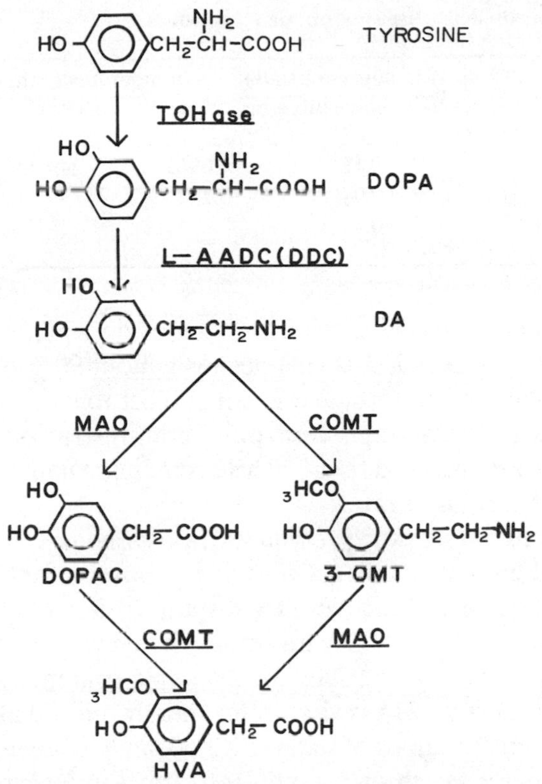

Figure 3.1 Synthesis and catabolism of dopamine. Dietary tryrosine is hydroxylated in the ring-3 position by tyrosine hydroxylase enzyme (TOHase), to yield 3,4 dihydroxyphenylalanine (DOPA). The terminal carboxy group of DOPA is then removed by L-aromatic acid decarboxylase (L-AADC), also known as DOPA-decarboxylase (DDC) enzyme, to yield dopamine (DA). Intraneuronal DA catabolism involves as the first step oxidation by monoamine oxidase (MAO) enzyme to yield dihydroxyphenylacetic acid (DOPAC). Methylation of DOPA at the ring-3 hydroxyl group by catechol-O-methyl transferase (COMT) enzyme yields homovanillic acid (HVA) and is believed to occur primarily in nonneuronal (i.e., glial) compartments. A small fraction (about 20%) of DA catabolism also begins in glial compartments with methylation by COMT enzyme to yield 3- methoxytyramine (3-OMT) followed by MAO-catalyzed oxidation to HVA.

and 30MT is a substrate for MAO; the final common reaction product is homovanillic acid (HVA).

DOPAC and HVA are large organic acids which can be actively transported across the brain-blood barrier by a probenecid-sensitive carrier. Thus, the rise in brain and/or spinal fluid DOPAC and HVA levels following probenecid administration provides an estimate of dopamine turnover (synthesis) rate. Likewise, measurement of brain tissue (DOPAC +

Table 3.3 ^{3}H-Cocaine Binding and Dopamine (DA), DOPAC, and HVA
Levels in Parkinson's Disease Putamen Specimens*

	(pmol/gram tissue)	(nanograms/gram tissue)		
	^{3}H-Cocaine blinding	DA	DOPAC	HVA
Control	0.124	2696.	249	5962
PD	0.049	113.	36	1665
(% Control)	40.	4.2	14	28

*Data derived from reference 28.

HVA)/(DA) ratios provides a relative index of dopaminergic neuronal
activity. Normally, this ratio is small, because about 90% of striatal DA
exists in vesicular storage form and is not subject to catabolism. During
pharmacological stress (e.g., reserpine administration) or loss of
dopamine neurons, this ratio rises because remaining neurons synthesize
and release DA at a faster rate.

DA is also conserved by the presynaptic nerve endings from which it is
released. A sodium-dependent active transport system for DA is located
on the nerve endings and removes DA at submicromolar concentrations
from the synaptic cleft. This DA transport system can be inhibited by a
variety of drugs including cocaine, and available evidence suggests that
this "newly transported" DA is also preferentially utilized in neurotrans-
mission. Low concentrations of radioactive cocaine incubated with brain
tissue homogenates attach preferentially to this DA transport site. Cocaine binding has thus recently emerged as a biochemical probe to quan-
titate the loss of presynaptic dopaminergic nerve endings in postmortem
PD brain specimens [28].

Postmortem data from PD brain specimens reflect both the progressive loss of striatal DA and increase in apparent DA turnover as the disease progresses (see Table 3.1). Comparison of these human data (Table
3.1) with similar data from MPTP-treated primates (Table 3.2) reveals
striking correlations between those most severely affected with idiopathic
PD and primates with experiental parkinsonism. Lastly, recent measure-
ments of ^{3}H-cocaine binding to brain homogenates from idiopathic PD
patients demonstrate the utility of this technique for defining depletion
of striatal DA transport sites (Table 3.3).

How do the above data provide guidelines for rational DA replacement
with levodopa? Two related issues require discussion; these concern 1)
the entry of levodopa into brain tissue and conversion to DA, and 2) synaptic retention and utilization of DA derived from levodopa.

With regards to the first point, levodopa must pass three major tissue-compartment barriers (GI tract to blood, blood to brain extracellular fluid, and brain extracellular fluid to intraneuronal compartments) before synaptically relevant conversion to DA can occur. At each of these three barriers, L-dopa appears to be transported by carrier systems that exhibit similar substrate specificities for "large-neutral" amino acids. There is no evidence to suggest that dopaminergic nerve endings transport levodopa any more or less efficiently than do nondopaminergic nerve endings.

Several recent studies have demonstrated the influence of plasma amino acid concentrations on the ability of exogenous levodopa to improve clinical symptoms of PD patients. Experimentally induced increases in plasma large neutral amino acid levels block striatal accumulation of radioactive levodopa in controls [19] and markedly worsen PD symptoms in patients with advanced disease receiving intravenous levodopa infusions [23]. These studies support attempts to improve the response to levodopa therapy by avoiding mealtime dosing and large amounts of protein.

The metabolism of levodopa in the brain depends mainly upon the presence or absence of DDC activity. As previously discussed, the majority (about 80%) or striatal DDC activity resides in dopaminergic nerve endings. The remainder (about 20%) is most likely located in intrinsic striatal neurons [21]. With progression of PD and increasing loss of striatal DA nerve endings, decarboxylation of levodopa to DA occurs to a greater extent in nondopaminergic compartments. The DA thus formed no longer has access to physiological DA storage mechanisms (vesicles and active transport system) and is retained in the striatum only briefly [29]. It is likely that these progressive reductions in the ability to synthesize and store DA derived from levodopa are partially responsible for the appearance of shortened response times to levodopa therapy as PD progresses [29].

DOPAMINE RECEPTORS: DIRECT AGONIST THERAPY

Postsynaptic Receptors

Following nerve terminal depolorization, DA is released by a calcium-dependent process, diffuses across the synaptic cleft, and binds reversibly to DA recognition sites on postsynaptic receptors. DA-receptor pharmacology has expanded significantly in the last decade. It now appears as though there are at least two major subtypes of postsynaptic DA receptors in the brain: D-1 and D-2 [31]. These subtypes vary both in the drug specificity for agonists and antagonists of their recognition sites and the effects of agonist binding upon activation or inhibition of cyclic nucleotide second messenger systems.

The D-1 DA receptor subtype is activated by DA and selectively by SKF 38393, blocked selectively by SCH 23390 and not by many traditional neuroleptic drugs (e.g., chlorpromazine, haloperidol), and is positively linked to the adenylate cyclase second-messenger system. Thus, the DA-stimulated adenylate cyclase system in striatal homogenates is mediated by D-1 receptors. D-2 DA receptors are activated by DA and selectively by the ergoline LY 141865 and the ergot pergolide, blocked potently by many neuroleptic drugs (haloperidol, chlorpromazine), and are negatively coupled to the adenylate cyclase system.

D-1 and D-2 DA receptors overlap extensively in their anatomic distribution and appear to be located primarily on intrinsic striatal neurons and nerve endings in substantia nigra derived from striatal neurons. Although D-2 DA receptors appear to mediate many of the behavioral effects of neuroleptic drugs, the functional role of D-1 receptors is not yet clear. Using behavioral tests to discriminate D-1 from D-2 effects has shown few differences in animals with intact dopaminergic innervation of and normal DA levels in the striatum. If the dopaminergic innervation of the striatum is surgically interrupted or if DA levels are pharmacologically reduced, then separable D-1 and D-2 receptor-mediated effects are more clearly observed. These animal experiments have yielded inconsistent data about which DA receptor subtype (if either) is primarily responsible for modulating motor function. As an example, in MPTP-induced parkinsonism in primates, D-1 agonist administration fails to correct the motor abnormalities whereas D-2 agonist treatment relieves the parkinsonian symptoms [10]. However, in reserpine-treated rats, simultaneous D-1 and D-2 agonist treatment appears necessary to correct fully the akinesia arising from DA depletion [13]. It is likely that D-1 and D-2 receptors interact in an as yet unknown fashion to control motor function. To what extent striatal D-1 versus D-2 receptor activation is responsible for the beneficial effects of exogenous levodopa in human PD remains to be elucidated.

Presynaptic Receptors

DA-utilizing neurons in the substantia nigra and closely adjacent midbrain ventral tegmental area possess receptors on their cell bodies (soma) and dendrites that recognize DA and DA agonists. These presynaptic DA receptors, also referred to as *autoreceptors* or *somatodendritic receptors* regulate DA neuronal firing rates by monitoring DA release after neuronal depolarization. Activation of presynaptic DA receptors by released DA or exogenous DA agonist decreases DA neuronal firing rate, thus serving as a local regulatory feedback system for modulating dopaminergic tone in the striatum.

DA agonists clinically useful in treating PD interact potently with presynaptic and postsynaptic DA receptors. The pharmacological profile of DA presynaptic receptors is similar to postsynaptic DA receptors of the D-2 subtype. Thus, pergolide and LY 141865 are similar in potency to DA and more potent than bromocriptine; the selective D-1 agonist SKF 38393 is only weakly active at presynaptic DA receptor site [33].

The functional implication of presynaptic DA receptor existence in treating PD is not clear. In advanced PD, almost all substantia nigra DA neurons have degenerated, and few presynaptic DA receptors remain. However, in early PD, DA agonist interaction with presynaptic receptors on surviving zona compacta neurons could theoretically be deleterious to treatment. In this situation, DA agonists would be predicted to decrease the firing rates of surviving DA neurons and worsen PD symptoms. To date, the DA agonist most frequently utilized as initial therapy for early PD symptoms is bromocriptine. The low potency with which bromocriptine activates presynaptic DA receptors [33] may be fortuitous in preserving its efficacy in early PD. However, some clinical experience has indicated that low bromocriptine doses worsen PD symptoms in moderately affected patients [30].

NONDOPAMINE NEUROTRANSMITTER ALTERATIONS IN PD

Norepinephrine

The locus ceruleus neurons in the brainstem comprise the other major pigmented nuclear group in the mammalian brain and are the source of forebrain innervation by norepinephrine-utilizing terminals. The neurons in the locus ceruleus frequently show depigmentation, reduction in number, and Lewy bodies in PD brains. Pronounced loss of forebrain DA and pigmented zona compacta neurons is always found in PD, but pathological involvement of the locus ceruleus is more variable and is reflected in heterogeneity of norepinephrine (NE) depletion. While, reductions in forebrain NE levels and DBH activity have been reported in PD brain by several investigations [17], the degree of reduction rarely exceeds 50% of age-matched controls.

Several recent studies suggest that sudden "off" swings or freezing spells, more common in later stages of PD, may be due to NE deficiency. This idea is based on studies by two groups [6,22] that have shown that akinesia/freezing spells are ameliorated by administration of 3,4 dihydroxyphenylserine (DOPS), the immediate amino acid precursor of NE, which is converted to NE by DDC. However, not all investigators have found DOPS to be helpful in PD patients affected with akinesia [25,32].

Serotonin (5-HT)

The forebrain's innervation by 5-HT is derived from neurons of the raphe nuclei located in the midline of the midbrain. There is no consistent neuropathological involvement of the raphe group in PD, although serotonin is consistently diminished throughout the forebrain in postmortem PD specimens [17]. This reduction probably arises from a functional alteration in raphe neuronal activity in PD. There is evidence in animals of a functional interaction between raphe and locus ceruleus neurons. Whether the alterations in NE metabolism discussed above are related to decreased 5-HT levels in PD is not clear.

Gamma-Aminobutyric Acid (GABA)

GABA is a four-carbon amino acid derived from the decarboxylation of L-glutamic acid by the enzyme glutamate decarboxylase (GAD). GABA is the major inhibitory neurotransmitter of the mammalian forebrain and is utilized by 25-40% of forebrain synapses, depending on the region examined. Its ubiquitous occurrence in millimolar concentrations in gray matter guarantees its involvement in virtually all forebrain activities. Deficits of GABA function are of pathophysiological significance in experimental epilepsy [26] and Huntington's disease [20], conditions where loss of GABA-utilizing neurons has been unequivocally demonstrated.

Animal studies have shown that GABA-utilizing striatal and substantia nigra (zona reticulata) projection neurons mediate the motor behaviors brought about by drug stimulation of striatal DA receptors [3]. Thus, GABA activity is critically involved in maintaining striatal output after administration of dopamimetic drugs. Because GABA levels rise rapidly following death, determination of postmortem tissue GABA concentrations

Table 3.4 Glutamic Acid Decarboxylase (GAD) Activities in Parklnson's Disease Basal Ganglia*

Brain region	Percent control GAD (means ± S.E.M.)
Caudate	46 ± 9 (5)**
Putamen	55 ± 8 (7)
Globus pallidus	41 ± 9 (3)
Substantia nigra	32 ± 4 (7)

*Data derived from references quoted in 3.
**Number in parentheses is the number of separate
   studies.

is of limited value. Rather, most investigators have relied on measuring GAD activity, which appears to have much better postmortem stability.

A summary of the available literature on GAD determinations in PD basal ganglia specimens reveals a consistent trend of GAD reduction (Table 3.4) The degree of GAD reduction is greatest in the substantia nigra and approaches that found in Huntington's disease. Because of the critical importance of substantia nigra GABA function in transmitting striatal DA activity, the marked reduction of nigral GAD in PD may be responsible for part of the progressive resistance to dopamimetic therapy in advanced PD. These findings led to a preliminary trial of concomitant GABA-mimetic therapy in patients resistant to levodopa, with encouraging results [4]. It is possible that concomitant GABA-mimetic therapy will improve the responses of patients with advanced PD to dopamine agonist therapies.

Acetylcholine (ACh)

Striatal acetylcholine is localized primarily in intrinsic cholinergic interneurons, and there is no pathological evidence for loss of these interneurons in PD. ACh is synthesized from choline and acetyl-CoA by the enzyme choline acetyltransferase (CAT), and ACh levels decline very rapidly following death. CAT activity and localization by immunohistochemical methods serve as markers for cholinergic interneurons. The reductions in striatal CAT activity found in PD specimens [17] probably reflect functional alterations in cholinergic neuronal activity rather than primary pathological events.

On other forebrain regions, ACh derives in large part from neurons located in a diffuse nuclear group located at the base of the forebrain, the nucleus basalis of Meynert. These neurons decline in number with normal aging but are severely depleted in dementing illnesses such as Alzheimer's disease. PD patients with significant dementia at death have increased loss of these basal forebrain cholingeric neurons compared to nondemented PD controls [34]. This finding is consistent with reports of reduction of cerebral cortical and hippocampal CAT activity levels in some PD specimens [27] and suggests that two separate neurodegenerative disorders (PD and Alzheimer's disease) can coexist in the same patient.

FREE-RADICAL SCAVENGING SYSTEM ABNORMALITIES IN PD

Free radicals are highly reactive chemical species with unpaired electrons that are constantly being formed in multiple biological processes. Commonly occurring free radicals such as peroxide, superoxide, and hydroxyl are formed during the oxidation of biogenic amines including dopamine. If not deactivated, free radicals are capable of damaging important cellular components such as membrane lipids and DNA. Brain tissue normally contains enzymes such as catalase, glutathione peroxidase, and superoxide dismutase, which are responsible for scavenging endogenously produced free radicals and preventing neuronal damage.

Recent data suggest that the substantia nigra may be particularly vulnerable to the effects of free radical formation, and that such free radical formation within the pigmented dopaminergic zona compacta neurons may be partially responsible for the normal age-related decline in compacta neuron number [12,24]. It is therefore of great interest that PD substantia nigra specimens show marked reduction in superoxide dismutase activity and nearly total loss of glutathione (a necessary substrate for glutathione peroxidase) [24]. Such findings have prompt-ed the hypothesis that therapy with antioxidant agents such as MAO inhibitors, vitamin C (ascorbic acid), or vitamin E (tocopherol) may retard the decline in compacta dopamine neuron number associated with progression of PD.

REFERENCES

1. Ballard PA, Tetrud JW, Langston JW: Permanent human parkinsonism due to 1-methyl-4-phenyl-1,2,3,6-tetrahydropyridine (MPTP): seven cases. Neurology 35:949-956, 1985.
2. Bannon MJ, Goedert M, Williams B: The possible relation of glutathione, melanin and 1-methyl-4-phenyl-1,2,5,6-tetrahydropyridine (MPTP) to Parkinson's disease. Biochem Pharmacol 33:1697-1698, 1984.
3. Bennett JP Jr, Ferrari MB, Cruz CJ: GABA-mimetic drugs enhance apomorphine-induced contralateral turning in rats with unilateral nigrostriatal dopamine dener-

vation: implications for the therapy of Parkinson's disease. Ann Neurol 21:41-45, 1987.

4. Bergmann KJ, Limongi JCP, Lowe Y-H et al: Progabide in decompensated Parkinson's disease: implications of dopaminergic-GABAergic interaction for levodopa-induced fluctuations. In Usdin E (ed): Catecholamines: Part B: Neuropharmacology and Central Nervous System-Therapeutic Aspects. New York, Alan R. Liss, 1984, pp 53-60.

5. Bernheimer H, Birkmayer W, Hornykiewicz O et al: Brain dopamine and the syndromes of Parkinson and Huntington. Clinical, morphological, and neurochemical correlations. J Neurol Sci 20:415-455, 1973.

6. Birkmayer W, Birkmayer L, Lechner H, and Riederer P: DL:-3,4- threo DOPS in Parkinson's disease: Effects on orthostatic hypotension and dizziness. J Neurol Trans 58:305-313, 1983.

7. Bunney BS: The electrophysiological pharmacology of midbrain dopaminergic systems. In Horn AS, Kork J, Westerink BHC (eds): The Neurology of Dopamine. New York, Academic Press, 1979, pp 417-452.

8. Burns RS, LeWitt PA, Ebert MH et al: The clinical syndrome of striatal dopamine deficiency. Parkinsonism induced by 1-methyl-4- phenyl-1,2,3,6-tetrahydropyridine (MPTP). New Engl J Med 312:1418-1421, 1985.

9. Chiveh CC, Burns RS, Maubey SP et al: Current concepts III. Primate model of parkinsonism: selective lesion of nigrostriatal neurons by 1-methyl-4-phenyl-1,2,3,6-tetrahydropyridine produces an extrapyramidal syndrome in rhesus monkeys. Life Sci 36:213-218, 1985.

10. Close SP, Marriot AS, Pay S: Failure of SKF 38393-A to relieve parkinsonian symptoms induced by 1-methyl-4-phenyl-1,2,3,6-tetrahydropyridine in the marmoset. Br J Pharmacol 85:320-322, 1985.

11. Davis GC, Williams AC, Markey AP et al: Chronic parkinsonism secondary to intravenous injection of meperidine analogues. Psychiatry Res 1:249-254, 1979.

12. Freeman BA, Crapo JD: Biology of disease: free radicals and tissue injury. Lab Invest 47:412-426, 1982.

13. Gershanik O, Heikkila RE, Duvoisin RC: Behavioral correlations of dopamine receptor activation. Neurology 33:1489-1492, 1983.

14. Hassler R. Zur pathologic der paralysis agitaons und des postenzephalitischen Parkinsonismus. J fur Psychologie und Neurologie (Leipzig) 48:387-476, 1938.

15. Hornykiewicz O: Die Tipische Lokalisation und das verhalten von noradrenalin und dopamin (3-hydroxytyramin) in der substantia nigra des normalen und parkinsonkranken menschen. Wiener Klinische Wochenschrift 75:309-312, 1963.

16. Hornykiewicz O: Dopamine (3-hydroxytyramine) and brain function. Pharmacol Rev 18:925-962, 1966.

17. Javoy-Agid F, Rubert M, Taquet H, et al: Biochemical neuropathology of Parkinson's disease. In Hassler RG, Christ JF (ed): Advances in Neurology 40:189-198. New York, Raven Press, 1984.

18. Langston JE, Forno LS, Rebert CS, Irwin I: Selective nigral toxicity after systemic administration of 1-methyl-4-phenyl-1,2,5,6-tetrahydropyridine (MPTP) in the squirrel monkey. Brain Res 292:390-394, 1984.

19. Leenders KL, Poewe WH, Palmer AJ, et al: Inhibition of L-[^{18}F]- fluorodopa uptake into human brain by amino acids demonstrated by positron emission tomography. Ann Neurol 20:258-261, 1986.

20. McGeer PL, McGeer EG: Enzymes associated with the metabolism of catecholamines, acetylcholine and GABA in human controls and patients with parkinson's disease and Huntington's chorea. J Neurochem 26:65-76, 1976.

21. Melamed E, Hefti F, Pettibone DJ, et al: Aromatic L-amino acid decarboxylase in rat corpus striatum: implicaitons for action of levodopa in parkinsonism. Neurology (NY) 31:651-655, 1981.

22. Nauabayaski H: Pharmacological basis of akinesia in Parkinson's disease. J Neurol Trans Suppl 19:143-151, 1983.

23. Nutt JG, Woodward WR, Hammerstad JP, et al: The "on-off" phenomenon in Parkinson's disease. Relation to levodopa absorption and transport. N Engl J Med 310:483-488, 1984.

24. Perry TL, Godiz DV, Hansen S: Parkinson's disease: a disorder due to nigral glutathione deficiency? Neurosci Letters 33:305-310, 1982.

25. Quinn NP, Perlmutter JS, Marsden CD: Acute administration of DL-threo-DOPS does not affect the freezing phenomenon in parkinsonian patients. Neurology 34:149A, 1984.

26. Roberts E: Failure of GABAergic inhibition: a key to local and global seizures. In Delgado-Escueta AV, Ward, Jr. AA, Woodbury DM, Porter RJ (eds): Basic Mechanisms of the Epilepsies-Molecular and Cellular Approaches. New York, Raven Press, 1986, pp 319-341.

27. Ruberg M, Poska A, Javoy-Agid F, Agid Y: Muscarinic binding and choline acetyltransferase activity in parkinsonian subjects with reference to dementia. Brain Res 232:129-139, 1982.

28. Schoemaker H, Pimoule C, Arbilla S, et al: Sodium dependent [^{3}H] cocaine binding associated with dopamine uptake sites in the rat striatum and human putamen decrease after dopaminergic denervation and in Parkinson's disease. Naunyn-Schmied Arch Pharmacol 329:227-235, 1985.

29. Spencer SE, Wooten GF: Altered pharmacokinetics of levodopa metabolism in rat striatum deprived of dopaminergic innervation. Neurology 34:1105-1108, 1984.

30. Stern MB, Vernon GM, Gollomp SM, Hurtig HI: Low-dose, slow- increase bromocriptine in patients with progressive Parkinson's disease and complications of levodopa therapy. Bull Clin Neuroscience, 51:52-56, 1986.

31. Stoof JC, Kababian JW: Two dopamine receptors: biochemistry, physiology, and pharmacology. Life Sci 35:2281-2296, 1984.

32. Suzuki T, Sakoda S, Veji M, et al: Treatment of parkinsonism with L-threo-3,4-dihydroxyphenylserine. Neurology 34:1446-1450, 1984.

33. White FJ, Wang RY. Pharmacological characterization of dopamine autoreceptors in the rat ventral tegmental area: microiontophoretic studies. J Pharmacol Exp Ther 231:275-280, 1984.

34. Whitehouse PJ, Hedreen JC, White CL III, Price DL: Basal forebrain neurons in the dementia of Parkinson disease. Ann Neurol 13:243-248, 1983.

35. Wilson SAK: Progressive lenticular degeneration: a familial nervous disease associated with cirrhosis of the liver. Brain 34:295-489, 1912.

II
Treatment of Early
Parkinson's Disease

Chapter 4

The Drug Therapy of Early Parkinson's Disease*

C. D. Marsden

SPECIFIC ANTIPARKINSONIAN DRUGS fall into two classes. First there are those that are modestly effective but relatively easy to use, with a more or less standard dosage schedule and well-defined side effects; for example, anticholinergics and amantadine. Second, there are the more powerful drugs, requiring more complicated dosage and producing greater side effects; for example levodopa and bromocriptine.

Today, most patients with Parkinson's disease present with mild to moderate disability. The problems discussed in this chapter include: which of these drugs to use, what dosages to use, and when to employ them in the treatment of early Parkinson's disease.

WHY IS THERE A PROBLEM?

The reason there is no clear answer to the question is that adequate clinical trials have not been undertaken. There are historical and practical reasons for this.

When levodopa was introduced into routine clinical practice in the 1960s, every neurologist had a large pool of patients with Parkinson's disease to treat. Clinical trials of levodopa were easy to arrange. The next years were spent discovering the problems of long-term levodopa ther-

---

* This chapter is based upon a lecture given at the First Annual Parkinson's Disease Symposium in Bermuda in October 1985, and at a meeting in Oxford in March 1986. The latter is to be published in *More Dilemmas in Neurology,* (edited by C. Warlow and J. S. Garfield). I am grateful to these editors for permission to reproduce this revised paper here.

apy, and trying to find means to overcome them. Only when it became apparent that levodopa was not going to be the complete answer to treating this condition did attention turn to alternative strategies.

By then, however, the number of patients available for testing new approaches to treating the de novo case had fallen dramatically. The incidence of Parkinson's disease is nearly 20 cases per 100,000 per year [18]. An average District Hospital population in the United Kingdom will generate some 40 to 60 new cases of Parkinson's disease a year. Perhaps a third of these patients are not referred to a hospital for some years until problems in treatment arise. Of those that are, most will have been started on treatment by their general practitioner, and at least half will be sent to geriatricians. Thus, a neurologist who wants to study the treatment of de novo cases may see no more than 20 new patients a year, of which most already will be on treatment. Larger numbers may be collected from a wider geographical area, but problems arise in conducting long-term clinical trials where travel to a hospital is difficult.

The need for multi-center clinical trials has only recently been appreciated by those who work in the field of Parkinson's disease. The problems are considerable. Quite apart from difficulties in adequate interrater reliability for instruments to assess efficacy, the numbers required to detect differences between treatment schedules are formidable. To detect a 10% difference between two drugs may require around 1,000 de novo cases. Trials may need to be continued for 5 or more years if important long-term benefits are to be established.

However, despite the difficulties, the problems are not insurmountable. A number of multicenter trials have been set up throughout the world to answer the questions discussed in this chapter, but the results will not be known for some time.

WHEN TO START TREATMENT?

When Should One Start Some Form of Drug Treatment?

Anticholinergics, amantadine, bromocriptine and levodopa are not thought to slow or prevent the progression of the underlying pathology of Parkinson's disease. When these drugs are stopped, the patient relapses back to a state of parkinsonism at least as bad and often much worse than before treatment was started. The pathological changes in the brains of patients dying with Parkinson's disease look no different from those seen before the advent of drug therapy.

Conventional drug treatment today is thought to be a substitution treatment for striatal dopamine deficiency (like insulin for diabetes) rather than a cure. So treatment is required only when disability warrants it. Indeed, the whole management of Parkinson's disease hinges upon the individual patient's disabilities imposed by their illness in relation to their needs—in other words, their handicaps. Drug therapy should be tailored to try to overcome the handicap in each individual.

This means that drug treatment in the earliest stages of the disease may not be required at all. Only when the handicap is evident is therapy indicated.

What About Deprenyl?

The statements given above may not cover the drug deprenyl (or selegiline). One of the outcomes of the remarkable MPTP story is that inhibition of monoamine oxidase B by a drug such as deprenyl may slow progression of Parkinson's disease.

The story goes like this [19]. MPTP, a contaminant of certain "designer drug" substitutes for morphine and heroin, produces dramatic parkinsonism in man and non-human primates. Young drug addicts exposed to MPTP rapidly develop a parkinsonism that, in virtually all respects, resembles idiopathic Parkinson's disease in the middle-aged or elderly. MPTP itself is not toxic in animals, but requires conversion to MPP+, the agent that destroys the substantia nigra. MPTP conversion to MPP+ is achieved by monoamine oxidase B. MPTP toxicity in animals can be prevented by pretreatment with deprenyl (or other monoamine oxidase B inhibitors). So, if idiopathic Parkinson's disease is due to exposure to something like MPTP in the environment, for which there is no concrete evidence, then deprenyl might prevent progression of the disease.

All this is hypothesis, but Birkmayer and colleagues [1], in a retrospective analysis of patients treated or not treated with deprenyl, claim that those on deprenyl live a few years longer than those not so treated? There are reservations about these data (retrospective analysis, different levodopa dosage in the two groups, selection of patients for deprenyl treatment, and so on), but the suggestion is there, and many patients know about it via the media and lay societies.

The story does not end there. The toxin MPP+ selectively kills nigral neurons because it is taken up into those cells via the dopamine uptake mechanism, where it is trapped by neuromelanin. Dopamine uptake blockers, such as mazindole and benztropine, can prevent MPTP toxicity in animals. Once in substantia nigra neurons MPP+ may eventually kill them by the generation of free radicals. Free radical scavengers such as vitamins C and E, glutathione and so on, may protect against MPTP toxicity.

So now there are many suggestions for trying to prevent the progression of Parkinson's disease; for example, deprenyl, mazindole, and free radical protective agents. All are under clinical trial, but results will take many years to obtain.

Meanwhile, what advice should be given to patients? Ideally, all de novo cases should enter one of these clinical trials. However, where that is not feasible, I would apt for giving deprenyl to de novo patients on diagnosis, in the slight hope that it might help to slow disease progression. Deprenyl has been used for many years in Europe as an adjunct to levodopa therapy (inhibition of monoamine oxidase B potentiates and slightly prolongs the duration of action of a dose of levodopa), so we know its relative safety and mild side effects.

When Should Levodopa be Started?

This is a controversial issue, but the debate is not as polarized as it might appear [4,11,15]. There are theoretical reasons, but little practical evidence [6] to fear that levodopa might be harmful. levodopa administration might, for instance, increase the formation of toxic free radicals and oxygen species in remaining dopaminergic neurons, which already are at such risk due to their neuromelanin-synthetic systems. These are only theoretical reasons for concern, but it does seem prudent not to jump into levodopa therapy from the start.

There is, however, another reason for such caution. Loss of efficacy of levodopa therapy occurs in a substantial proportion of patients on chronic treatment, often due to the emergence of fluctuations in response, and unpleasant side effects such as dyskinesias and psychiatric complications. Fluctuations in response with dyskinesias appear in around 50% of cases after 5 years of treatment, and in nearly all after 10 years. Our own data and that of others (see below) suggest that the prevalence of dyskinesias and fluctuations increases progressively with the duration of levodopa treatment. As a result, a decline in benefit occurs with time, and this generally is independent of the stage of disease severity or the duration of the disease at the time treatment is commenced.

This leads to the suggestion that one should reserve the undoubted benefits of levodopa for that period of life when they are most needed.

However, there are some who believe that the response to levodopa is less satisfactory if given later in the illness (see below), and that the drug should be employed early in the disease.

The proponents of early treatment claim that loss of benefit during long-term levodopa therapy is unrelated to duration of treatment, but is rather a function of the severity and duration of the disease before levodopa is started. Markham and Diamond [10] in a paper titled "Evidence to Support Early Levodopa Therapy in Parkinson's Disease," felt that their data indicated that long-term disability depended upon duration of disease before treatment was started, rather than upon duration of treatment. This led them to suggest that "delaying therapy fails to improve disability in the early years of disease and does not confer any benefit in later years...Our data support the benefits of beginning levodopa therapy early." Their conclusion, however, was not as controversial as one might suppose: "We suggest that the proper time is when an adequately informed patient is willing to start a medicine that must be taken many times a day for years, which needs frequent adjustments of dosage, which very often causes troublesome but not life-threatening side effects, but which may extend the quality and span of life to a normal range." Recently, these authors have reanalyzed their data after a longer period of follow-up; their original findings were confirmed [12]. Hoehn [5] also concluded that postponing levodopa treatment increased the proportion of patients who became unresponsive, and that delaying therapy did not confer any future benefit.

The proponents of delayed treatment, however, suggest that their data indicate that loss of benefit is related to duration of treatment, rather than to duration of disease or its severity before therapy is begun.

Most observers agree that the *initial therapeutic* response to levodopa treatment is not greatly influenced by the degree of disability when drug therapy is commenced [6,7,21]. Certainly, those with mild to moderate severity improve to the same extent, and even those with severe disability often show considerable benefit. In addition, many clinicians have reported that the frequency of loss of response to long-term levodopa therapy is independent of disease duration but rather depends upon how long patients have received treatment [3,6,7,9,13,14,21]. The general view is that the factors responsible for loss of response, including the emergence of fluctuations, dyskinesias and dementia, increase in prevalence with the duration of levodopa treatment.

A dispassionate view of these opposite conclusions is that they are not the extreme positions that they may appear to be at first sight. What is at issue is how to treat patients with Parkinson's disease today. Markham and Diamond's data was based on careful follow-up of a cohort of patients started on treatment when levodopa first became available. Many of these patients had severe disease of long duration. Their data was based on comparison of three groups: those treated with levodopa within 1 to 3 years of disease onset, those treated within 4 to 6 years, and those treated within 7 to 9 years. Nowadays most patients require levodopa within a few years of onset of the disease, and no neurologist would withhold levodopa until the patient is severely disabled.

I therefore take the view that levodopa therapy should be reserved for when it is needed. This reintroduces the crucial notion of handicap as the guiding principle in the drug management of Parkinson's disease. To emphasize the point, take four examples:

1. A 40-year-old, mildly affected individual with a stable job, whose employers are prepared to continue his work, perhaps at a less demanding level, and whose financial status would not suffer too much. Such a patient might opt for a long-term view by taking amantadine and/or an anticholinergic to begin with, keeping levodopa in reserve for later years.
2. A 50-year-old, more severely affected, whose work is already at risk, with a family at school and heavy financial commitments. Early levodopa treatment may be required to keep the patient in employment.
3. A 60-year-old, happy to retire, with limited physical activities, may be quite adequately managed with amantadine for some years before levodopa is required.
4. A 70-year-old, active tennis player and "champion of industry," still with ambitions, may request early levodopa treatment, on the grounds of "a short life and a happy one."

The decision about when to start treatment in an individual patient and which class of drugs to use, thus revolves around assessing the patient's disability at that time, judging the patient's requirements and expectations now and for the future, and then discussing the pros and cons of the various options in order to arrive at an agreed decision. There is no single rule to govern this question; each patient's individual problem has to be considered on its merits.

A WORD ON AMANTADINE AND ANTICHOLINERGICS

If we accept that not everyone requires levodopa therapy from the beginning, it is necessary to consider the relative merits of the long-established anticholinergic drugs and the newer amantadine.

In recent years, I have become less enamored of anticholingerics. Undoubtedly they do exert a useful, if modest, antiparkinsonian action, and can be used successfully in the early stages of the illness. My worry concerns their potential long-term effects.

Unfortunately, a proportion (probably nearer to one fifth than to the usually quoted figure of one third) of patients with Parkinson's disease dement [2]. The biochemical basis of dementia in Parkinson's disease centers on Lewy body degeneration of neurons in the substantia innominata with consequent loss of cortical cholinergic projections (biochemically similar to the findings in Alzheimer's disease) [16]. Anticholinergic drugs might be expected to make this situation worse. Whether early anticholinergic treatment predisposes to later cortical cholinergic deficit and dementia is unknown, but the fear is there. For this reason I am now less keen to use anticholinergics, and certainly do not employ them in the elderly.

Accordingly, I favor amantadine for the newly diagnosed case who requires some therapy, but whose handicap does not warrant levodopa treatment. Amantadine possesses modest but definite antiparkinsonian action, and may prove adequate initially. Much has been written about the development of tolerance, or loss of benefit from amantadine. Undoubtedly this occurs, possibly as a result of progression of the disease, but a significant proportion of patients with early disease may be successfully managed on amantadine for years.

LEVODOPA OR BROMOCRIPTINE?

A relatively new debate is whether bromocriptine is a better drug than levodopa to commence with, when handicap demands strong therapy (see Chapter 5).

The issue revolves around:

1. The evidence that dyskinesias and fluctuations are less prevalent in those started on bromocriptine alone, compared with those started on levodopa. From the limited number of studies available, this seems to be the case. For instance, in a recent investigation by Rinne [17], after 3 years of bromocriptine treatment, only 2 of 21 (10%) patients

had developed dyskinesias and none had fluctuations, against 57% and 19% respectively in 217 patients commenced on levodopa. Lees and Stern [8] provided similar data in an earlier study. Thus there might be advantages in the long-term of using bromocriptine rather than levodopa. However, this conclusion must be tempered by a second factor.

2. Only a relatively small proportion of patients can be managed on bromocriptine alone. Lees and Stern [8] found that only 11 of 50 patients commenced on bromocriptine alone were still on that regime 3 years later. Rinne [17] found that of 76 patients so treated, only 21 (28%) were on bromocriptine alone after 3 years of therapy. The remainder had stopped the drug because of an insufficient therapeutic response or distressing side effects. These data suggest that less than a third of de novo patients can be managed on bromocriptine alone. The rest require addition of levodopa to maintain benefit. Moreover, Lees and Stern [8] found that some patients requiring substitution of levodopa after starting on bromocriptine did not appear to respond as well as expected.

This evidence raises questions about the apparent lower incidence of dyskinesias and fluctuations in those started on bromocriptine compared with those commenced on levodopa. The figures for frequency of complications refer to those who could be managed on bromocriptine for years, and ignores the two thirds or so who could not. It is quite possible that this minority who could manage on bromocriptine represent a subgroup less prone to develop complications of long-term treatment. Alternatively, they may require a relatively small dose of dopamine replacement therapy. There is no easy way to resolve these doubts.

A NOTE ON LOW-DOSE VERSUS HIGH-DOSE BROMOCRIPTINE

Teychenne and colleagues [20] have championed the view that adequate relief of parkinsonism can be achieved by using very small doses of bromocriptine, with small gradual increments over long periods of time, providing that one is patient. In principle, this is attractive, for the lower the dose, the less likely are side effects. Undoubtedly, some de novo patients may be managed successfully by this approach, but many cannot. This dilemma is more apparent than real, for the dose required varies from case to case, as with levodopa. In addition, the slower the introduction of bromocriptine, the longer it takes to achieve a response.

A PRACTICAL COMPROMISE

The present state of affairs appear to be:

1. Most patients cannot be managed on bromocriptine alone for any length of time.
2. However, chronic levodopa therapy carries a high risk of the emergence of disabling complications of long term treatment, namely dyskinesias and fluctuations.

A compromise is to use the two drugs together. By combining levodopa with bromocriptine one can keep the dose of levodopa low, thereby avoiding any (as yet unproven) long-term effects of the latter, as well as perhaps reducing the chances of subsequent development of dyskinesias or fluctuations.

Specifically, when the handicap warrants a powerful form of treatment, I start the patient on 100 mg levodopa with 25 mg carbidopa (Sinemet). I always start with this combination to ensure an adequate intake of the decarboxylase inhibitor to reduce the chances of initial nausea and vomiting. I titrate the dose of Sinemet to about 4 to 6 tablets daily (400 mg to 600 mg levodopa a day). Many patients respond adequately within this dose range. If they do not, or if they lose control, I then add bromocriptine, rather than increase the dose of levodopa further. The dose of bromocriptine is increased until adequate control is achieved.

There is some data to support this combined-treatment concept. Rinne [17] compared a group of patients treated with levodopa alone (217 cases) with another group treated with levodopa plus bromocriptine (42 cases). (It should be noted that this was not a prospective randomized clinical trial.) Patients were followed for 3 years, during which time bromocriptine was withdrawn in the combined group in 11 patients, and 3 other patients were lost to follow-up. Average levodopa dosage (in the form of Madopar) for those who continued treatment for 3 years in the former group was 798 mg/day (with decarboxylase inhibitor), in the latter group it was 660 mg/day plus 16.6 mg/day of bromocriptine. The overall clinical improvement achieved was comparable in the two groups (37% and 39% respectively). In terms of side effects, fluctuations in the levodopa group occurred in some 19% of patients over 3 years, compared with only 4% in those treated with combined levodopa and bromocriptine; dyskinesias occurred in 57% of those on levodopa, alone but in only 21% of those on combined therapy.

At the present time, this combined approach appears to be a reasonable compromise for management. To restate an earlier observation, such a conclusion is based upon inadequate data. We require well-designed clinical trials on large numbers of patients for an adequate length of time to prove whether this is indeed the best we can do with contemporary drugs.

REFERENCES

1. Birkmayer W, Riederer P: Deprenyl prolongs the therapeutic efficacy of combined L-DOPA in parkinson's disease. Advances in Neurology 40:475-481, 1984.
2. Brown RG, Marsden CD: How common is dementia in Parkinson's disease? Lancet 2:1262-1265, 1984.
3. Fahn S, Bressman SB: Should levodopa therapy for parkinsonism be started early or late? Evidence against early treatment. Can J Neurol Sci 2(suppl):200-205, 1984.
4. Hachinski V: Timing of levodopa therapy. Arch Neurol 43:407, 1986.
5. Hoehn MM: Parkinsonism treated with levodopa: progression and mortality. J Neurol Trans (Suppl 19):253-264, 1983.
6. Lees AJ: Is levodopa harmful? In: Warlow CP, Garfield JS (eds): Dilemmas in the Management of the Neurological Patient. London, Churchill Livingston, pp 115-125, 1984.
7. Lees AJ: levodopa treatment and Parkinson's disease. Quart J Med 59:535-547, 1986.
8. Lees AJ, Stern GM: Sustained bromocriptine therapy in previously untreated patients with Parkinson's disease. J Neurol Neurosurg Psychiat 44:1020-1023, 1981.
9. Lesser RP, Fahn S, Snider SR, Cote LJ, Isgreen WP, Barrett RE: Analysis of the clinical problems in parkinsonism and the complications of long-term levodopa therapy. Neurology 29:1253-1260, 1979.
10. Markham CH, Diamond SG: Evidence to support early levodopa therapy in Parkinson's disease. Neurology 31:125-131, 1981.
11. Markham CH, Diamond SG. Modification of Parkinson's disease by long-term levodopa treatment. Arch Neurol 43:405-407, 1986a.
12. Markham CH, Diamond SG. Long-term follow-up of early dopa treatment in Parkinson's disease. Ann Neurol 19:365-372, 1986b.
13. Marsden CD, Parkes JD: Success and problems of long-term levodopa therapy in Parkinson's disease. Lancet 1:345-349, 1977.
14. Marsden CD, Parkes JD: "On-off" effects in patients with Parkinson's disease on chronic levodopa therapy. Lancet 1:292-295, 1976.
15. Melamed E: Initiation of levodopa therapy in parkinsonian patients should be delayed until the advanced stages of the disease. Arch Neurol 43:402-405, 1986.
16. Quinn NP, Rossor MN, Marsden CD: Dementia and Parkinson's disease—pathological and neurochemical considerations. Br Med Bull 42:86-90, 1986.
17. Rinne UK. Combined bromocriptine-levodopa therapy early in Parkinson's disease. Neurology 35:1196-1198, 1985.
18. Schoenberg BS: The epidemiology of movement disorders. In: Marsden CD, Fahns S (ed): Movement Disorders II. London, Butterworth, 1986.
19. Snyder SH, D'Amato RJ: MPTP: a neurotoxin relevant to the pathophysiology of Parkinson's disease. Neurology 36:250-258, 1986.
20. Teychenne PF, Bergsrud D, Racy A, Elton RL, Vern B: Bromocriptine: low-dose therapy in Parkinson's disease. Neurology 32:577-583, 1982.
21. Yahr MD: Long-term levodopa therapy in Parkinson's disease. Lancet 1:706-707, 1977.

Chapter 5

Dopamine Agonists in Early Parkinson's Disease

C. Warren Olanow

THE INTRODUCTION OF LEVODOPA (L-DOPA) was a major therapeutic breakthrough, and it revolutionized the treatment of Parkinson's disease (PD) [6]. It provided clinical benefits and increased longevity for approximately 80% of PD patients. Dosage limitations related to gastrointestinal side effects were largely eliminated by combining levodopa with a peripheral decarboxylase inhibitor. However, chronic levodopa treatment is associated with a gradual loss of efficacy and the development of adverse reactions such as mental changes, dyskinesias, dystonias, and fluctuations in motor performance that include end-of-dose deterioration and the "on-off" phenomenon [22,34]. These motor fluctuations in PD were not seen prior to the introduction of levodopa, and studies now suggest that low-dose levodopa regimens are associated with a lower incidence of adverse reactions as well as with a longer latency until their development [27]. Thus there is concern that these adverse reactions are related to the cumulative dosage of levodopa employed. Mechanisms that may be responsible include alterations in dopamine receptor sensitivity and fluctuations in levodopa bioavailability due to competition with other amino acids for gastrointestinal absorption and transport into the central nervous system [24]. Additionally, free radicals and other metabolites generated by levodopa metabolism may contribute to dopamine neuronal damage. Once adverse reactions and loss of efficacy develop, current thera-

Presynaptic Neuron:
Levodopa, a metabolic precursor of dopamine,
undergoes decarboxylation to dopamine in the
presynaptic neurons originating in the substantia nigra.

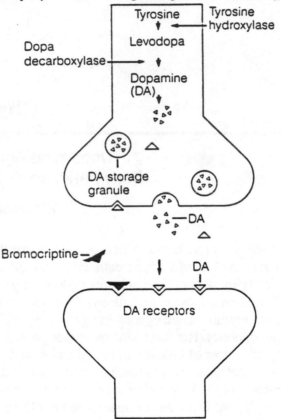

Postsynaptic Neuron:
DA receptors can be stimulated by DA or by
direct-acting DA agonists, such as bromocriptine that
bypass the presynaptic neuron.

Figure 5.1 The pre- and post-synaptic dopamine neuron.

pies are often unsatisfactory, and interest has focused on alternative
methods of treating PD patients early in their course in an effort to prevent the development of adverse reactions and to slow down the rate of
disease progression. One such method is the use of a group of drugs
known as dopamine agonists.

DOPAMINE AGONISTS

Dopamine agonists are a diverse group of structures with differing physical and chemical properties. They have in common a dopamine-like moiety within their molecular structure that allows for direct stimulation of the postsynaptic dopamine (DA) receptor. They differ from conventional treatment with levodopa, which has to be taken up into the terminals of the nigrostriatal DA neurons, converted to DA by a decarboxylase enzyme, stored in vesicles and then released into the synaptic cleft in order to stimulate the postsynaptic DA receptors (Figure 5.1). Dopamine agonists bypass the degenerating nigrostriatal neurons, do not depend upon a pool of decarboxylase enzyme, and directly stimulate the postsynaptic dopamine receptor. Further, dopamine agonists are metabolized differently than is levodopa, thereby avoiding potentially toxic metabolites of levodopa [1,2].

Two different types of DA receptors have been identified—a D-1 and D-2 receptor [16]. The D-1 receptor is characterized by its linkage with adenylate cyclase; the D-2 receptor is characterized by a high affinity for neuroleptics. The D-1 and D-2 receptors appear to exist in both low- and high-affinity states. Levodopa stimulates both D-1 and D-2 receptors. Dopamine agonists have varying receptor stimulation profiles and may have agonist or antagonist properties for either the D-1 and D-2 receptors. The theoretical advantages of dopamine agonists are illustrated in Table 5.1.

Most, but not all dopamine agonists are natural or synthetic derivatives of ergot alkaloids. Because of their alpha-adrenergic properties, ergots have been primarily used in the treatment of migraine headache and as inducers of uterine contraction. In the middle 1800s, ergot derivatives were employed in the treatment of PD, but were found to be relatively ineffective [3]. These ergots, however, were of low molecular weight and

Table 5.1 Theoretical Advantages of Dopamine Agonists

1. Direct stimulation of the postsynaptic dopamine receptor, thereby bypassing the degenerating nigrostriatal neuron.
2. Independent of the pool of decarboxylase enzyme necessary for conversion of levodopa to dopamine.
3. More stable compounds with longer half-lives.
4. Avoid pharmacokinetic problems associated with levodopa.
5. Varying profiles of dopamine receptor subset stimulation.
6. Avoid potentially toxic by-products of levodopa metabolism.

are now appreciated to have subclinical therapeutic activity. In 1954, it was demonstrated that some ergot alkaloids inhibit prolactin secretion by stimulating dopamine receptors in the pituitary gland [31]. Subsequently apomorphine, a dopamine agonist, was shown to have antiparkinsonian properties and to have an effect even during akinetic or "off" episodes, thus illustrating that dopamine receptors may retain the capacity to respond during clinical fluctuations [5].

A variety of dopamine agonists have now been tested in clinical trials, using prolactin inhibition as a screen for compounds with potential antiparkinsonian efficacy [23]. Bromocriptine mesylate (Parlodel) has been the most widely studied dopamine agonist [20]. Bromocriptine is an ergot alkaloid (a synthetic lysergic acid aminopeptide) that has a low affinity for alpha-adrenergic receptors, thus making it largely devoid of vasoconstricting properties. It is a potent D-2 receptor agonist and mildly antagonizes the D-1 receptor—a different pattern of receptor subset stimulation than that of levodopa. It is rapidly absorbed from the gastrointestinal tract, but 94% undergoes first-pass metabolism in the liver. Its plasma half-life of 7 hours is approximately 4 times that of levodopa and twice that of levodopa/carbidopa. Pergolide mesylate, a semisynthetic ergoline derivative, is another D-2 receptor agonist that has been widely studied and demonstrated to have potent antiparkinsonian activity [32]. It differs from bromocriptine in that it is more potent, has a longer half-life, and mildly stimulates the D-1 receptor. Other dopamine agonists that have been used in the treatment of PD but that are not currently available in the United States include lisuride, lergotrile, mesulergine, ciladopa, and terguride. A number of other dopamine agonists are currently under investigation in the laboratory and in preliminary clinical trials.

When bromocriptine was first introduced, attempts were made to use it as a substitute for levodopa in patients with advanced PD. Very high doses had to be employed, resulting in numerous side effects; and, if it was effective at all, the benefit was short lived. Consequently, bromocriptine is no longer utilized in this fashion. Subsequently, bromocriptine was employed as an adjunct to levodopa therapy for patients with increasingly disability who had developed adverse reactions [10,15,21]. In general, studies demonstrated that approximately 50% of these patients improved when bromocriptine was added to their levodopa regimen. In a study of patients with Stage 3 and Stage 4 PD, Hoehn and Elton noted that the addition of bromocriptine results in improvement in the total PD score and a reduction in adverse reactions when compared with placebo controls [14]. Relatively high doses of bromocriptine were required in this patient population to produce clinical benefit, resulting in a relatively high incidence of side effects including psychosis, orthostatic hypotension, nausea, vomiting, and peripheral edema [17]. Dose-related reactions severe enough to necessitate withdrawal from medication have been reported in up to 58% of patients. Further although clinical benefits may be statistically significant, they are not attained in all patients, and the level of clinical improvement in many instances does not translate into a meaningful reduction in functional disability.

DOPAMINE AGONISTS AS PRIMARY TREATMENT FOR PARKINSON'S DISEASE

The major drawback of levodopa is that it provides only temporary relief of symptoms. A large number of patients go on to develop drug-induced side effects that are often as debilitating as the symptoms of the disease itself. Once these adverse reactions have developed, the addition of dopamine agonists may be of value, but combination treatment is generally less than satisfactory. The mechanism leading to these adverse reactions is unknown, but levodopa itself has been implicated in their pathogenesis. Rajput et al., in a retrospective analysis, demonstrated that adverse reactions occurred with a greater frequency and a shorter duration when patients took higher doses of levodopa [27], suggesting that the development of adverse reactions was related to the cumulative dose of levodopa taken by patients during the course of treatment. It has also been demonstrated that complications associated with long-term levodopa therapy occur sooner when levodopa is combined with a peripheral decarboxylase inhibitor from the onset of therapy [7]. The finding that adverse reactions occurred with reduced frequency when low doses of levodopa were employed [19] led to strategies in which attempts were made to further reduce the cumulative levodopa dose by initiating therapy with dopamine agonists. When bromocriptine was employed as initial therapy in these previously untreated PD patients, the incidence of adverse reactions was extremely low and in some studies nonexistent. Rascol et al., using a mean dosage of 56.5 mg of bromocriptine per day, reported that no patient developed dyskinesia, dystonia or motor fluctuations after 4 to 8 years of treatment [28]. Lees and Stern similarly showed a low incidence of adverse effects using bromocriptine alone in previously untreated PD patients [18]. These studies, however, were retrospective and because a prospective, randomized controlled trial has not been done, it is possible that patients using bromocriptine had milder disease compared with those using levodopa. There is a tendency to adminster levodopa more readily in rapidly advancing disease in nonrandomized studies. To try to overcome the deficiencies of retrospective analysis, prospective studies have been designed in which previously untreated PD patients were randomized to treatment with either levodopa or bromocriptine and followed by blinded observers. In such a study performed at our institution, we employed the lowest doses of levodopa or bromocriptine that would provide an adequate antiparkinsonian response and carefully monitored the clinical response, and, the incidence and severity of adverse reactions [25]. Forty-seven patients who were randomized as part of this study have now been followed for a mean of 2-1/2 years. Adverse reactions have been more common in levodopa-treated patients; 2 have developed motor fluctuations and 9 have experienced peak-dose dystonia. Adverse reactions were much less common in bromocriptine-treated patients, none of whom experienced motor fluctuations. Only 1 patient had mild peak-dose dystonia. Patients continue to be monitored as part of this ongoing study, but in general we have been impressed by the relatively mild nature of side effects in both treatment groups. We suggest that this is related to minimizing the cumulative levodopa dosage, either by withholding levodopa or employing the drug in the lowest dose that provides a satisfactory clinical response. Bromocriptine side effects have largely been eliminated by employing low-dose regimens, and no patient has withdrawn from this study because of drug-related side effects. Clinical benefits were comparable in both treatment groups for the first 6 months [26], but were longer lasting in levodopa-treated patients than in those randomized to receive bromocriptin (Figure 5.2). Open retrospective studies by Rinne have corroborated these findings [29,30]. He documented a markedly reduced incidence of adverse reactions in patients treated with bromocriptine monotherapy, but found that the majority eventually needed adjunctive treatment with levodopa. Studies employing pergolide and lisuride as the initiating dopamine agonist have yielded similar results. Long-term prospective multicenter double-blind studies are currently underway, but it would appear that although dopamine agonists are associated with a reduced incidence of adverse reactions, clinical benefits are short lived. Monotherapy with currently available dopamine agonists does not provide satisfactory long-term treatment for the majority of PD patients.

COMPARISON OF % IMPROVEMENT IN TOTAL PARKINSON SCORE

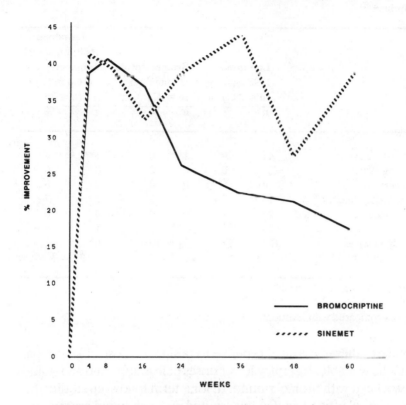

Figure 5.2 Comparison of percentage of improvement in total Parkinson score in untreated Parkinson patients randomized to treatment with either bromocriptine or Sinemet

DOPAMINE AGONISTS IN EARLY COMBINATION WITH LEVODOPA

It thus appears that we have a dilemma. Levodopa provides a better antiparkinsonian response, whereas dopamine agonists are associated with fewer adverse reactions. Rinne noted that patients treated with levodopa had antiparkinsonian responses that persisted during 3 years of treatment, but that were associated with a high incidence of adverse reactions. On the other hand, patients initiated on treatment with bromocriptine had fewer adverse reactions but did not sustain their antiparkinsonian response (Table 5.2). To deal with this problem he proposed the early combination of levodopa with dopamine agonists [29]. He introduced levodopa therapy, and then employed bromocriptine as an adjunct early

Table 5.2 Parkinson Disability and Adverse Reactions During Treatment of Parkinson Patients with Levodopa, Bromocriptine or Combined Levodopa and Bromocriptine*

Variables	Levodopa (798 mg/day) (n = 217)		Bromocriptine (28 mg/day) (n = 21)		Levodopa (660) mg/day)† bromocriptine (16.6 m/day) (n = 28)	
	n	%	n	%	n	%
Disability						
End-of-dose disturbances	41	19	1**	0	1**	4
Early morning akinesia	22	10	0	0	0	0
Nocturnal akinesia	14	6	0	0	0	0
Freezing episodes, random	16	7	1	5	2	7
Freezing, episodes, dose- related	24	11	0	0	0	0
Dystonia	36	17	0**	0	1	4
Peak-dose dyskinesias	123	57	2†	10	6†	21
Improvement of PD (%)	37 = 1		15 = 3†		39 = 3	

*Adapted from Rinne, reference 29.
**$p < 0.05$
†$p < 0.001$ as compared with levodopa

in the course of therapy as an alternative to raising the dose of levodopa. In this way, he was able to employ lower doses of levodopa and avoid side effects associated with bromocriptine. In long-term follow-up studies, he noted that clinical efficacy in patients treated with combined bromocriptine and levodopa was comparable to that attained with levodopa alone and superior to that with bromocriptine alone. Motor fluctuations and peak-dose dyskinesias were less frequently associated with combined therapy than with levodopa alone. He concluded that combined therapy offered the advantages of the superior clinical effectiveness of levodopa and the reduced incidence of fluctuations and dyskinesias afforded by dopamine agonists. These benefits have persisted during the course of 5 years of follow-up [30].

To accomplish these results, Rinne initiated treatment with levodopa and used bromocriptine as an adjunct. These same results have been attained in our studies by initiating therapy with a dopamine agonist and employing levodopa as an adjunct when the clinical effectiveness of the agonist wears off. This approach may have the additional benefit of delaying the introduction of levodopa if in fact the benefits of combined therapy are related to a reduction in total cumulative levodopa dosage. Using this approach and employing doses of levodopa of approximately 350 mg per day, we have as yet observed no end-of-dose deterioration or dyskinesia in patients who have been followed for up to 3 years.

Numerous studies have now demonstrated the potential advantages of employing combined levodopa/dopamine agonist therapy early in the course of treatment [12,33], and at the present time combined therapy appears to be the preferred method of treating early PD. We have recommended the following principles in initiating therapy:
1. Delay the introduction of dopamine-replacement therapy until patients have developed functional disability.
2. Use the lowest dosage of levodopa that will provide an acceptable clinical response.
3. Use a dopamine agonist such as bromocriptine as an adjunct to levodopa therapy early in the course of treatment, prior to the development of adverse reactions, as an alternative to raising the levodopa dosage.

The above approach could be modified by initiating therapy with a dopamine agonist and using levodopa as an adjunct, as discussed above. Studies comparing the relative benefits of these two approaches are underway, but it is not clear at present that there is an advantage of one over the other. Anticholinergic agents and amantidine (Symmetrel) may be useful in this population of patients as a means of delaying the introduction of dopamine-replacement therapy when symptomatic treatment becomes necessary.

We favor initiating therapy with the lowest dose of drug that provides an adequate antiparkinsonian response. We have noted that patients who initially fail respond to a given dose may develop clinical improvement if maintained on the same dosage for a period of time. We therefore do not encourage rapid dosage changes in these patients. We introduce levodopa in the form of Sinemet with 1/2 of a 25-100 tablet per day. The daily dose is then increased by 1/2 tablet no more frequently than once a week until the desired clinical response is attained. If a satisfactory response has not been obtained with a dose of 300 mg to 400 mg per day of levodopa in the form of Sinemet, a dopamine agonist—bromocriptine or pergolide—is combined with levodopa. Bromocriptine is initiated at a dose of 1.25 mg per day, and the daily dose is increased by 1.25 mg no more frequently than once a week. Using this approach, approximately 80% of newly diagnosed PD patients who are capable of responding can be adequately managed without adverse reactions during the first 3 to 5 years of therapy using doses of levodopa and bromocriptine not exceeding 400 mg and 20 mg, respectively. In this respect, it is important to keep in mind that patients with Parkinson-plus syndromes (progressive supranuclear palsy, olivopontocerebellar atrophy, Shy-Drager syndrome, striatonigral degeneration, etc.) may initially present with features suggestive of PD (see Chapter 1). These patients typically do not respond to dopamine-replacement therapy, and failure to develop an adequate clinical response using the above regimen might indicate that the patient has a Parkinson-plus syndrome. It now appears that these conditions are more common than was initially appreciated and constitute up to 20% of all patients presenting with parkinsonism.

RATIONALE FOR COMBINED THERAPY

One can only speculate as to why combined therapy appears to offer advantages in comparison with treatment with levodopa or with dopamine agonists alone. Most thinking has centered around a reduction in the cumulative dose of levodopa consumed by a patient over the course of treatment. Levodopa and dopamine are oxidized by a monoamine oxidase B to form hydrogen peroxide (H_2O_2). H_2O_2 is in turn oxidized to form the hydroxyl free radical. Free radicals contain an unpaired electron spinning in orbit. This is an unstable state and results in these free radicals reacting vigorously with a variety of chemical compounds, including proteins, DNA, and lipids, causing damage to these structures. The hydroxyl free radical is one of the most potent of the free radicals and is capable of generating considerable cellular damage. Under ordinary circumstances, the body has defense mechanisms to protect against the formation of free radicals. This is primarily accomplished by the "scavenger" enzymes, which include glutathione peroxidase, catalase, and superoxide dismutase. If the body's defense mechanisms are inadequate to control free radicals, either because of a reduced number of scavenger enzyumes or too much substrate, oxidative stress damage can result [13]. Therefore, the metabolism of dopamine as well as exogenous levodopa might result in nigral damage and worsening PD. Although it is not yet established that the scavenger-enzyme systems are deficient in patients with PD, there is recent information suggesting that levodopa administration can result in oxidation stress and tissue damage through the accumulation of the oxidized form of glutathione (GSSG), even in the absence of the formation of hydrogen peroxide [4]. Further, magnetic resonance imaging and chemical analyses have demonstrated increased iron in the substantia nigra of patients with PD and in the putamen of patients with Parkinson-plus syndromes [8]. Iron may simply be a marker of the degenerative process, but it is noteworthy that iron is a transition metal and is capable of delivering an electron to oxygen or hydrogen peroxide, thus facilitating oxidation reactions and the development of free radicals [13]. For these reasons, a rational argument can be advanced to support the use of low-dose levodopa.

There is also evidence to suggest that dopamine agonists and levodopa are mutually enhancing. Dopamine receptor stimulation by dopamine agonists may be diminished by pretreatment with alpha-methylparatyrosine, which inhibits the synthesis of dopamine [9]. This suggests that dopamine formed in the presynaptic neuron enhances the therapeutic efficacy of bromocriptine. Further, most available dopamine agonists primarily stimulate the D-2 receptor and have little if any effect on the D-1 receptor. Stimulation of the D-1 receptor by dopamine, however, might provide additional benefit in PD patients treated with dopamine agonists. Thus combined therapy allows for D-2 receptor stimulation by dopamine agonists plus levodopa-induced D-1 receptor stimulation. A pure D-1 receptor agonist is presently being investigated and has been reported to have some antiparkinsonian effect in animal models. Human studies to test the combined efficacy of D-1 and D-2 receptor agonists are anxiously awaited.

It is also possible that dopamine agonists such as bromocriptine enhance the effect of levodopa on the D-2 receptor. Receptor studies indicate that D-1 and D-2 receptors exist in both a low- and high-affinity state for dopamine stimulation. Goldstein has proposed that bromocriptine may induce receptor changes that enhance the effect of levodopa administration [20].

Finally, one has to consider the possibility that dopamine agonists may protect nigral neurons from degeneration. At the present time this is only a theoretical consideration, but Felton and coworkers at the University of Rochester have demonstrated that the addition of pergolide to the diet of rats protects against the age-related decline of dopaminergic neurons in the substantia nigra [11].

SUMMARY

Current treatment for PD remains primarily symptomatic, and levodopa remains the drug of choice. Long-term administration of levodopa, however, is associated with loss of efficacy and the development of motor fluctuations and dyskinesias. Initiation of treatment with dopamine agonists has been demonstrated to be associated with a reduced incidence of fluctuations and dyskinesias, but clinical benefits are not long-standing. Now the use of combined therapy early in the course of treatment seems to provide PD patients with the best chance of obtaining a long-lasting response without the development of later problems. Although it has not yet been established, it is suspected that adverse reactions correlate with a loss of dopamine neurons and progression of PD, and that they may be associated with the cumulative dose of levodopa administered during treatment. Combined therapy allows for a reduction in the total cumulative levodopa dosage, which may represent the basis for the beneficial effect of this approach. There is considerable interest in studies trying to define the role of antioxidant therapies and neurotransplantation as more definitive forms of treatment for PD; however, combined therapy using low doses of levodopa and a dopamine agonist early in the course of therapy is currently the recommended treatment for patients with PD.

REFERENCES

1. Calne DB: Dopaminergic agonists in the treatment of Parkinsonism. Clin Neuropharmcol 3:153-166, 1978.
2. Calne DB, Burton K, Beckman J, Martin R: Dopamine agonists in Parkinson's disease. Can J Neurol Sci 11:221-224, 1984.
3. Charcot JM: Lecons sur les maladies du systeme nerveux faites a la Salpetriere. Recueillies et publiees par Bourneville a Paris. Delahaye et Lecrosnier, pp 155-158, 1892.
4. Cohen G: Personal communication, 1987.
5. Cotzias GC, Papavasilou PS, Tolasal ES, Mendez JS, Bell-Midulla M: Treatment of Parkinson's disease with aporphines—possible role of growth hormone. N Engl J Med 294:567-572, 1976.
6. Cotzias GC, Van Woert MH, Schiffer LM: Aromatic amino acids and modification of Parkinsonism. N Engl J Med 276:374-379, 1967.
7. De Jong GJ, Meerwaldt JD: Response variations in the treatment of Parkinson's disease. Neurology 34:1507-1509, 1984.
8. Drayer BP, Olanow CW, Burger P, Johnson GA, Herfkens R, Riederer S: Parkinson Plus syndrome: Diagnosing using high-field imaging of brain iron. Radiology 159:493-498, 1986.
9. Duvoisin RC, Heikkila RE, Manzino L: Pergolide induced circuling in rats with 6 hydroxy dopamine lesions in the nigro-striatal pathway. Neurology 32:1387-1391, 1982.

10. Fahn S, Cote LJ, Snider SR: The role of bromocriptine in the treatment of Parkinsonism. Neurology 29:1077-1083, 1979.
11. Felten DL, Felten SY, Romano T, Wong D, Schmidt MJ, Clemens JA: Pergolide slows age-related changes of DA-continuing cells of the nigro-striatal system in Fischer 344 rats. Archives of Neurology, in press.
12. Fischer PA, Przuntek H, Majer M, Welzel D: Combined treatment of early stages of Parkinson's syndrome with bromocriptine and levodopa: a multi-center evaluation. Deutsch Med J 109:1279-1283, 1984.
13. Halliwell B, Gutteridge JMC: Oxygen radicals and the nervous system. TINS 22-26 Jan 1985.
14. Hoehn MM, Elton RL: Low dosages of bromocriptine added to levodopa in Parkinson's disease. Neurology 35:199-206, 1985.
15. Jansen NII: Bromocriptine in levodopa response losing Parkinsonism: a double-blind study. Eur Neurol 17:92-99, 1978.
16. Kebabian J, Calne D: Multiple receptors for dopamine. Nature 277:93-96, 1979.
17. Larsen TA, Newman RP, Lewitt PA, Calne DB: Bromocriptine dosage and the severity of Parkinson's disease. Neurology 31:662-667, 1983.
18. Lees AJ, Stern GM: Sustained bromocriptine therapy in previously untreated patients with Parkinson's disease. J Neurol Neurosurg Psychiat 44:1020-1023, 1981.
19. Lees AJ, Stern GM: Sustained low dose levodopa therapy in Parkinson's disease. A 3-year follow-up. Adv Neurol 37:9-15, 1983.
20. Lieberman A and Goldstein M: Bromocriptine in Parkinson's disease. Pharmacological Reviews 37:217-227, 1985.
21. Lieberman AN, Kupersmith M, Neophytides A: Bromocriptine in Parkinson's disease: report on 106 patients treated for up to 5 years. In Goldstein M (ed): Ergot Compounds and Brain Function; Neuroscience and Neuropsychiatric Aspects. New York, Raven Press, pp 45-53, 1982.
22. Marsden CD, Parkes JD: "On-off" effects in patients with Parkinson's disease on chronic levodopa therapy. Lancet 1:292-295, 1976.
23. Muller EE, Panerai AE, Cocchi D, et al: Endocrine profile of ergot alkaloids. Life Sci 21:1545-1558, 1977.
24. Nutt JG, Woodward WR, Hammerstad JP, Carter JH, Anderson JL: The "on-off" phenomenon in Parkinson's disease: Relation to levodopa absorption and transport. N Engl J Med 310:483-488, 1984.
25. Olanow CW, Alberts M: Low dose bromocriptine in previously untreated Parkinson patients. In Fahn S, Marsden D, Jenner P, Teychenne P (eds): Recent Developments in Parkinson's Disease. New York, Raven Press, pp 315-321, 1985.
26. Olanow CW, Alberts M, Staijch J, Burch G: A randomized blinded study of low dose bromocriptine versus low dose carbidopa-levodopa in untreated Parkinson patients. In Fahn S, Marsden CD, Calne D, Goldstein M (eds): Recent Developments in Parkinson's Disease vol 2. Florham Park, N.J.: MacMillan Health Care pp 201-208, 1987.
27. Rajput AH, Stern W, Laverty WH: Chronic low-dose levodopa therapy in Parkinson's disease. Neurology 34:991-996, 1984.

28. Rascol A, Montastrue JL, Guiraud-Chaumeil B, Clanet M: Bromocriptine as the first treatment of Parkinson's disease. Long-term results. Revue Neurologique 138:401-408, 1982.
29. Rinne UK: Combined bromocriptine-levodopa therapy early in Parkinson's disease. Neurology 35:1196-1198, 1985.
30. Rinne UK: Early combination of bromocriptine and levodopa in the treatment of Parkinson's disease: a 5-year follow-up. Neurology 37:826-828, 1987.
31. Shelesnyak MC: Ergotine inhibition of deciduoma formation and its reversal by progesterone. Am J Physiol 179:301-304, 1954.
32. Tanner CM, Goetz CG, Glantz RH, Glatt SL, Klawans HL: Pergolide mesylate and idiopathic Parkinson's disease. Neurology 32:1175-1179, 1982.
33. Teychenne PF, Bergsrud D, Racy A, Elton RL, Vern B: Bromocriptine: Low-dose therapy in Parkinson's disease. Neurology 32:577-583, 1982.
34. Yahr MD: Limitations of long-term use of anti-Parkinson drugs. Can J Neurol Sci 11:191-194, 1984.

Chapter 6

The Comprehensive Approach to Parkinson's Disease

Gwyn M. Vernon and Matthew B. Stern

PATIENTS WITH PARKINSON'S DISEASE experience not only physical changes but psychological ones as well. Responsibilities of dealing with a chronic disease for both the patient and family are never-ending. Daily attention must be focused on the subjective and objective symptoms, as successful adaptation patterns and healthy coping strategies are developed. As Parkinson's disease progresses slowly and insidiously, the patient and family gradually mobilize through several well-defined stages:

1. Confronting the reality of having a chronic illness.
2. Identification of problem areas and initiation of adaptation strategies.
3. Emergence of successful coping mechanisms, participation in therapy and an acceptance of Parkinson's disease as a partner in one's life [4].

The ease of adjustment to Parkinson's disease will be influenced by those interpersonal, environmental, and illness-related factors in the patient's and family's life. Age, personality, intelligence, self-care skills, values, beliefs, cognitive capacity, and the presence of a functional support network as well as access to health care services are important factors that will influence the adjustment to chronic illness [4].

This chapter discusses both the social and emotional problems that Parkinsonian patients and their families encounter in the course of disease, the stages through which patients and families evolve in their adaptation to Parkinson's disease, and the comprehensive approach necessary for successful care.

CONFRONTATION WITH THE REALITY OF HAVING A CHRONIC ILLNESS: THE EMOTIONAL RESPONSE

The variety of emotions accompanying the diagnosis of Parkinson's disease is vast. Patients and families may feel trapped in a maze of negative emotions including denial, anxiety, fear, hostility, regression, dependence, and depression. Physicians and health care providers must recognize the emotional impact of this chronic disease in order to develop a comprehensive care approach to patient care.

Denial

Initially, the patient may deny the diagnosis and search for other opinions and further medical testing. If the disease is in its early stages, a patient may choose to ignore both the symptoms and the urging of family members to seek medical care. Stress and tension can aggravate symptoms, frequently causing the early stage patient to attribute symptoms to nervousness or anxiety. Unrealistic hope is also a form of denial, as the patient bargains with himself, blaming his symptoms on imagination.

Anxiety and Fear

Anxiety and fear are common in early Parkinson's disease. Fear may in part be related to a lack of patient education at the onset of the disease. Many people remember an affected acquaintance or relative whose Parkinson's disease progressed relentlessly during the pre-levodopa era. Moreover, reaction to the diagnosis of Parkinson's disease may be colored by fears of losing independence and being a burden to others. The realization that preconceived life plans and hopes for the future will change dramatically can be devastating and result in grieving for the loss of one's former self. These feelings of grief, anxiety, and fear may resurface throughout the course of Parkinson's disease, particularly during periods of increased symptoms, gradual deterioration, or when medication is inadequately controlling the symptoms. Commonly, concurrent illnesses such as colds and urinary tract infections can temporarily exacerbate parkinsonian symptoms, causing fear of sudden disease progression.

Hostility

Hostility may be directed at health professionals or at well-meaning family members, and can take the form of mistrust or the inappropriate expression of anger.

Regression and Dependence

Patients may begin to make childlike demands on spouses and family members and react to new situations with emotional immaturity. Family members, in an effort to protect the patient, may assume responsibilities, rendering the patient more dependent than motor symptoms warrant. Although not necessarily harmful in the initial period of confirmed diagnosis, these patterns of behavior can be counterproductive to independent living and to the successful adjustment to a chronic disorder.

Depression

Depression can be a powerful, immobilizing emotion in many patients with Parkinson's disease (see Chapter 9). Depression may be a reaction to the initial diagnosis or evolve as lifestyle adjustments are imposed by the disease. The severity of depression is not necessarily related to the degree of motor impairment and may precede the onset of motor symptoms.

IDENTIFICATION OF PROBLEM AREAS

As the reality of Parkinson's disease becomes a fact of everyday living, patients and families will need to identify problem areas in their lives and develop strategies to cope with necessary changes. Common areas of concern include: the patient's self-esteem and changes in image, role changes within the family, issues of employment and finances, social isolation, sexuality, disease fluctuations, and caregiving decisions.

Self-Image and Change

Aging transforms the physique and influences the self-image. A loss of subcutaneous fat, atrophy of muscles, skin dryness, increased angularity of the body, and a stooped posture all contribute to the aged appearance. Parkinson's disease accentuates these changes in self-image. Persistent tremor and dyskinesias may cause weight loss, which can be aggravated by difficulties with cutting food, chewing, and swallowing. Furthermore, anorexia is a frequently encountered side effect of antiparkinsonian medication. A stooped posture, masked facies, and slowness in all movements may give a patient the appearance of exaggerated aging, whereas postural instability and muscle rigidity mimic the slow, stiff movements of elderly people.

Self-Esteem

Chronic illness is accompanied initially by a deterioration in self-esteem, as well as in physical strength and endurance. Altered physical reserves and a change in roles can put the patient in a vicious cycle of inactivity and lack of confidence [4].

Role Change

Parkinson's disease imposes role changes on the patient and family. Most people assume at least three simultaneous roles in their lives—as employee, parent, child or sibling. The more important these roles are to one's self-esteem and sense of stability, the more devastating role changes can be for affected patients.

Employment

Parkinson's disease is called a disease of the elderly, however, the onset of symptoms usually occurs in one's 50s and 60s. Many patients are still actively employed or perhaps beginning to consider retirement. The current median age of retirement is 62 years of age [8], and many Parkinsonians worry about their ability to fulfill job tasks that will be required until then. Patients may note a decline in their work performance, and may compensate by working longer hours and during weekends and vacations to catch up, thus causing stress at home. Moreover, job-related anxiety can exacerbate physical symptoms. In some cases, continued employment may be impossible, and the patient must take disability leave or early retirement.

Financial Problems

Financial problems are almost predictable for many patients. Income-producing skills may be altered, and disability payments, saving funds, and pensions may be limited. In addition to the loss of income, the family budget may be strained by medical expenses, especially expensive antiparkinsonian medications.

Medications can range from $25 to $700 a month, depending on the drugs necessary for effective treatment. Prescription plans that are available during the working years for many employees often cease upon disability or retirement. A recent survey of 100 patients revealed that less than 20% had a paid or partially reimbursed prescription plan [9].

In addition to antiparkinsonian medications, the cost of physician visits, home care, day care, and nursing care can be overwhelming. Even though some of these costs are covered by Medicare, Medicaid and private insurers, home care and nursing care is covered on an intermittent basis for skilled-level services only. The cost of private registered nurses and therapists can range from \$20 to \$50 per hour, while nurse's aides may cost \$7 to \$10 per hour. These are prohibitive sums for most patients. Third-party payers categorically do not reimburse for custodial care (bathing, feeding, transferring, companionship, toileting) at home, in a day care facility, or in a nursing home.

Social Isolation

Chronic diseases, especially those that impede mobility, cause social isolation. Parkinson's disease may cause difficulty driving a car or traveling on public transportation. Communication with others on the telephone may be strained by changes in voice volume and clarity. Disengagement from social contacts may be accentuated if the patient is embarrassed or easily frustrated by his symptoms.

Family members may also find it difficult to maintain a normal social life if they are dependent on the patient to drive the car or to make social arrangements. If the parkinsonian requires a great deal of care, family members usually have no additional time or energy to maintain an active social life.

Fluctuations

In the early stages of Parkinson's disease, many patients enjoy complete symtomatic relief with medication. However, as the disease evolves, the effectiveness of medication usually diminishes. After several years of treatment, patients often experience treatment-related problems, including loss of medication effectiveness, dyskinesias, wearing-off or end-of-dose failure, and the on-off phenomenon (see Chapter 7). In addition to understanding the medical aspects of these problems, the health care team must be aware of the psychological impact of complications of advanced disease. When loss of medication effectiveness occurs, patients may become anxious and fear progressive deterioration. Routine goals may become difficult to achieve, as patients experience difficulty in planning their activities during optimal medication effectiveness. Dyskinesias and fluctuations can be embarrassing for patients and may increase with stress, leading to fear and to withdrawals from new situations.

Care Decisions

Caregiving responsibilities are an important family consideration. Family caregivers may feel imprisoned and socially alienated by the daily patient care requirements. At the same time, however, they may have ambivalent feelings about seeking outside assistance—viewing it with guilt, as a symbol of their failure to cope with the home situation. Many families will dislike the lack of privacy when outside help is brought into the home, whereas others will be able to accept and enjoy the respite period.

It is within this framework of understanding the emotional as well as physical limitations of Parkinson's disease that a strategy for effective comprehensive care can evolve.

SUCCESSFUL COPING AND ADAPTATION STRATEGIES: THE COMPREHENSIVE APPROACH

It takes time for patients to adjust to the diagnosis of Parkinson's disease, and to learn how to cope with the multitude of problems they encounter. As the patient and family become more comfortable with the disease, they will actively participate with the health care team in order to solve specific problems as they arise. Open ongoing communication between the physician, patient, family, and other health care team members gradually evolves, while certain roles and responsibilities befall each member. This section discusses: 1) The role of patient, family, physician, nurse, and other health care professionals, and 2) The comprehensive or team approach to optimal Parkinson's disease management.

Role of the Physician

The physician is primarily responsible for an accurate diagnosis and for prescribing medications. He or she must lead the team of professionals providing comprehensive care to the parkinsonian patient and family, the components of which include:

1. Information and education.
2. Accessibility for personal and telephone consultations with patient and family.
3. Patient advocacy.
4. Prescribing ancillary services as needed (e.g., physical or speech therapy, counseling, or home care).

Office visits should include physical assessment, treatment, and education. Physicians should provide the patient and family with verbal and written information regarding the disease, its symptoms, the treatments, and expected outcomes of treatment. There are a variety of written materials available from the voluntary nonprofit organizations involved with Parkinson's disease for the physician to use in educating patients and families (see Appendix I). Sidney Dorros' book *Parkinson's: A Patient's View*

[2], and Dr. Roger Duvoisin's *Parkinson's Disease: A Guide for Patient and Family* [3] contain a wealth of information on the physical and emotional aspects of having Parkinson's disease (see Appendix III).

Patients and family members should be encouraged to telephone between physician visits if treatment is ineffective or when specific problems develop. These contacts are usually reassuring, if not always therapeutically rewarding. A policy of returning calls within 24 hours is usually satisfactory for handling nonurgent concerns relative to chronic disorders.

The physician must be prepared to be the patients' friend and advocate. Issues of employability or disability commonly arise. Many patients will request letters to assure the employer that they are capable of continued productivity. A letter describing the basics of Parkinson's disease, its symptoms, and how those symptoms interfere with the specific tasks at the workplace may help the patient stay employed. Questions about jury duty, driving, or traveling long distances must be addressed frequently.

Physicians must also make appropriate and timely decisions in choosing ancillary services, including nurses, social workers, physical, occupational and speech therapists. These services can be ordered by contacting the local hospital discharge planner or homecare department, a free-standing rehabilitation unit, or the local Visiting Nurse Association. Local information and referral centers for the American Parkinson Disease Association can also assist in finding appropriate resources (see Appendix II).

Nurses

Nurses traditionally provide acute care in hospitals, but with Parkinson's disease patients more commonly need nursing help outside the hospital. A patient at home can receive health assessments, medication instruction, and help with self-care by enlisting the services of a registered nurse. The community health nurse is often the coordinator of the outpatient health care program and the liaison between patient and physician.

Physical Therapy

The role of physical activity and exercise in Parkinson's disease is often underemphasized. The tendency of patients to become immobile should be counteracted with an appropriate daily maintenance-exercise program to avoid complications of immobility, such as pneumonia, constipation, venous stasis, and edema of legs. Although many patients will be capable of participating in active exercise such as swimming, jogging, or playing tennis and golf, others will require a program of gait training; balance, flexibility, stretching, and range-of-motion exercises; and safety instruction. The result in most cases is improved function and, perhaps most important, an enhanced sense of well-being. A physical therapist can tailor a program of exercise to the specific needs of the individual. When a cane or walker is needed, a physical therapist should instruct the patient directly on the proper use of these assistive devices.

Speech Therapy

Patients with Parkinson's disease usually experience problems with voice volume, clarity, initiation of speech, and swallowing. The services of a skilled speech therapist can improve the communication and swallowing problems of parkinsonians through exercises to control the rate and phrasing of speech, and to coordinate breathing with speaking and swallowing. Speech therapists can also advise patients on available amplification and communicative devices when needed.

Occupational Therapy

An in-home assessment of the patient by a skilled occupational therapist can lead to helpful instruction in the use of many assistive devices that can make activities of daily living easier.

Turning in bed can be enhanced by the use of a bed rail, bed pull, or trapeze. A stool beside the bed can ease the task of getting in and out of bed. Raising the toilet seat, placing a seat in the tub, and installing bathroom rails can assist the patient in toileting and bathing. Dressing can be aided by the use of button hooks, velcro clothing closures, or large zipper pulls. Built-up (weighted) eating utensils, scoop dishes, and plate guards are helpful for the patient who finds mealtime difficult. The occupational therapist can introduce a patient to many other community-available products that will enhance independence in the home environment (see Appendix III).

Counseling

Patients and family members are commonly overwhelmed by the physical and psychological adjustments that Parkinson's disease demands. Psychological counseling can be important to those in need. Counseling can be provided by a social worker, psychologist, or psychiatrist, depending on the complexity of the situation.

A clinical social worker or psychologist can provide counseling in adjustment skills. Locating and arranging helpful community resources such as day care, in-home care, or nursing homes is an important role of the social worker as the disease advances. A psychiatrist may be needed if the patient and/or family exhibit signs of major depressive disorders, or when a combination of psychotherapy and medication is warranted.

Role of the Patient and Family

The basic responsibilities of patients and families include:

1. To seek competent medical care.
2. To stay informed about Parkinson's disease.
3. To maintain one's worth and self-esteem [5,1].

The first responsibility of the patient and family is to establish a correct diagnosis. Twenty percent of patients referred to The Graduate Hospital Parkinson's Disease Center in Philadelphia do not have Parkinson's disease, but have rather another neurologic problem, such as essential tremor or one of the multiple system atrophies [7] (see Chapter 1). The diagnosis is the most important step toward appropriate management, because treatment and outcome are different for the specific neurologic disorders described.

When the diagnosis has been confirmed, patients and families should avail themselves of educational materials (see Appendix III), and learn what Parkinson's disease is and what it is not. A reasonable understanding of the illness, the treatment options available, and the goals of treatment should be sought. Patients who pursue unrealistic goals, such as a cure of the disease, will not fare as well physically or emotionally as those who learn the advantages and limitations of the available forms of treatment.

The third responsibility of the patient and family is to maintain the self-esteem of everyone involved with the disease. A strong support network of family members and friends is the most important asset for the patient and spouse in fulfilling the goal of realistic hope without false optimism. Patients should not alienate concerned loved ones, but include them in learning about and dealing with their neurologic disorder. Likewise, family members should assist the patient to maximize areas of remaining independence, and to avoid focusing on the worst disabilities. Because the natural progression of Parkinson's Disease is gradual and the rate is unpredictable, the majority of patients can participate in most activities for many years, gradually accommodating lifestyle to the degree of physical impairment.

Table 6.1 Parkinsonian Patient Profile*

Special attention: care provider

Factors especially pertinent to this patient are circled.

Parkinsonians may:

1. Choke on food!
   a. Be unable to feed themselves.
2. Develop pneumonia easily.
3. Have difficulty in communicating; low voice, slow to start speaking, mumble words. When rigid unable to press button to summon nurse.
4. Suffer from constipation.

5. Suffer from stress, which aggravates symptoms and creates more problems.
6. Be rigid or dyskinetic, and also be confused at times.

Precautions:

1. Make certain that food is in small pieces and has been swallowed.
2. Move patient every two hours.
3. Take time to listen; check patient as often as possible.

4. Patients need bulk in diet. Special foods to watch:
   a) Proteins-(quantity).
   b) Vitamin B-6 (foods to avoid or limit).
   c) Stool softener or laxative.

5. Patience and TLC are as essential as the medication.
6. It is vital that medicine be administered at the proper time *always!*

Additional problems

There is a special need for some manner of exercise every day.

Thank you for taking the time to understand my problem. You are keeping me alive!

---

*Reprinted with permission from Ida Raitano, the Parkinsonian Society of Greater Washington.

Sidney Dorros, in his book *Parkinson's: A Patient's View,* tells parkinsonians everywhere to "find a purpose in life, give and receive love, and have fun" [2]. The therapeutic effects of love and laughter have been well described by Sacks [6] and Dorros [2]. Emotional flexibility, a sense of humor, and above all, a sense of irony can reduce stress and tension in the struggle to cope with the vagaries of Parkinson's disease, in which emotional state mirrors motor dysfunction. Fun and recreation are vital pursuits in day-to-day planning.

Support Groups

Disease-related support groups came to life during the 1970s. Parkinson's disease has benefited from this revolution, with over 300 Parkinson's support groups in the U.S.A., England, Canada, and Japan. Support groups provide a forum for the exchange of information, discussion of conventional and experimental treatments, and peer emotional support.

Patients, family members, friends, and caretakers are the important players in the support-group drama. The range of activities include health education, social mixing, direct service to shut-ins, companion hours, assistance with shopping, friendly visitors, and telephone calls to the homebound.

The more creative groups have established such programs as weekly exercise groups, separate support groups for significant others, and group sessions for young or mildly impaired parkinsonians.

Advocacy for parkinsonians is extremely important and an activity essential to the core function of all support groups. An excellent example is the Parkinsonian Patient Profile developed by the Parkinsonian Society of Greater Washington (PSGW). This concise profile provides hospital staff with quick, easy-to-understand advice on caring for the hospitalized patient with Parkinson's disease (see Table 6.1).

SUMMARY

The comprehensive approach to Parkinson's disease entails a thorough understanding of a patient's reaction to chronic illness, and of problem areas that evolve with the (changing) symptoms of progressive disease. Optimal patient care requires a close working relationship among patient, family, physician, and other ancillary health care professionals. The successful adjustment to Parkinson's disease is dependent not only on medication, but on those services and support systems that provide emotional support and enhance independence and self-care.

REFERENCES

1. Cooper IR: Living with Chronic Neurologic Disease. New York, W.W. Norton, 1976.
2. Dorros S: Parkinson's: A Patient's View. Cabin John, MD, Seven Locks Press, 1981.
3. Duvoisin RC: Parkinson's Disease: a Guide for Patient and Family. New York, Raven Press (2nd Ed), 1984.
4. Miller JF: Coping with Chronic Illness. Philadelphia PA, F.A. Davis, 1983.
5. Parsons TE: Definition of Health and Illness in the Light of American Values and Social Structure. In Jaco EG (ed): Patients, Physicians and Illness. New York, The Free Press, pp 120-144, 1979.
6. Sacks O: Awakenings. Garden City, Doubleday, 1974.
7. Stern MB: Unpublished observations, 1986.

8. U.S. General Accounting Office Report: Retirement Before Age 65 is a Growing Trend in the Private Sector. July 15, 1985.
9. Vernon GM: Unpublished observations, 1986.

APPENDIX I

National Parkinson Organizations
- The American Parkinson Disease Association
  116 John Street
  New York, NY 10038
  1-800-223-APDA
- The American Parkinson Disease Association Information & Referral Centers
  Call 1-800-223-APDA for local centers
- National Parkinson Foundation, Inc.
  1501 N.W. 9th Avenue
  Miami, FL 33136
- Parkinson's Disease Foundation
  William Black Medical Research Building
  640-650 West 168th Street
  New York, NY 10032
- United Parkinson Foundation
  360 West Superior Street
  Chicago, IL 60610

National Parkinson Organizations/Support Groups
- Parkinson Support Groups of America
  11376 Cherry Hill Road #204
  Beltsville, MD 20705
- Parkinson's Educational Program (PEP)
  1800 Park Newport, Suite 302
  Newport Beach, CA 92660

APPENDIX II

Miscellaneous Resources

For Information on Resources in Your Community Contact:
- American Parkinson Disease Association
  Information & Referral Centers
  (Call 1-800-223-APDA)
- County Office on Aging
- Senior citizen centers
- Blue pages of the telephone directory, under heading *Health & Human Services*
- Social workers of the hospital or local Visiting Nurse Association (VNA)

For Physical, Occupational or Speech Therapy, Contact:
- Local hospital departments for outpatient use
- Visiting nurse associations
- Free-standing outpatient rehabilitation units

For Day Care and Respite Care Information, Contact:
- County office on aging
- Hospital social worker
- Visiting Nurse Association (VNA) social worker

For Local Support Group Information:
- The American Parkinson Disease Association 1-800-223-APDA
- Parkinson's Educational Program (PEP) 1-800-344-7872

APPENDIX III

A Guide for Patient and Family Reading

Cohlan, Alice R., Weiner, Florence D.: *Speech Problems and Swallowing Problems in Parkinson's Disease.* American Parkinson Disease Association, New York.

Cooper, I.R.: *Living with Chronic Neurologic Disease.* New York, W.W. Norton, 1976.

Dorros, Sidney: *Parkinson's: A Patient's View.* Cabin John, MD, Seven Locks Press, 1981.

Duvoisin, R.C.: *Parkinson's Disease: A Guide for Patient and Family.* New York, Raven Press (2nd edition), 1984.

Lavigne, Jeanne, Roberts, Kristine Mac: *Home Exercises for Patients with Parkinson's Diease.* American Parkinson Disease Association, New York.

Lieberman, A., Gopinathan, G., Neophytides, A., Goldstein, M: *Parkinson's Disease Handbook.* American Parkinson Disease Assocition, New York.

Pitzele, Sefra K.: *We are Not Alone: Learning to Live with Chronic Illness.* Thompson & Co., 1985.

Robinson, Marilyn B.: *Aids, Equipment and Suggestions to Help the Patient with Parkinson's Disease in the Activities of Daily Living.* American Parkinson Disease Association, New York.

III
Treatment of Advanced Parkinson's Disease

Chapter 7

Advanced Parkinson's Disease and Complications of Treatment

Howard I. Hurtig

MOST PATIENTS WITH PARKINSON'S DISEASE (PD) will eventually show evidence of motor deterioration, although the pace of the decline in function varies considerably among individuals. At the time of early diagnosis, especially in those with hemiparkinsonism, it is impossible to predict whether the disease will remain confined to one side indefinitely or will eventually become generalized. It is well to recall the clinical wisdom of William Gowers, an English neurologist, who in 1888 observed: "The variations in extension are thus so great as to make it difficult to foretell the course of a commencing case" [26].

Hoehn and Yahr [28] analyzed the clinical characteristics of a large population of parkinsonians at Columbia University's Neurological Institute during the 15 years just prior to the introduction of levodopa in the 1960s. The primary theme of their research was the natural history of PD and the associated risk of premature mortality. Hoehn and Yahr's conclusions were similar to those of Schwab [72] and Mjones [53], both of whom had previously documented the essential unpredictability of the course of the disease. Schwab found several clinical features to be unfavorable prognosticators: spread of symptoms from one side of the body to the other; the prominence of akinesia and hypophonic speech early in the evolution of the disease; and the appearance of dementia or cognitive dysfunction at any time. Hoehn and Yahr believed that a patient whose dominant symptom was tremor had a more benign course than a randomly chosen patient without tremor, but their attempts to correlate any cluster of signs or symptoms with ultimate outcome were unsuccess-

119

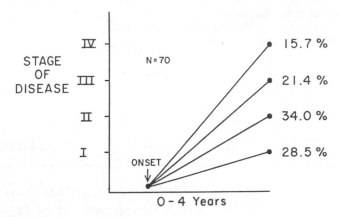

Figure 7.1 Variability of progression of the symptoms of PD (from Hoehn and Yahr [28]) among 70 patients observed for 4 years from onset. Stage of Disease is from the Hoehn and Yahr scale.

ful. People with onset of disease before age 50 tended to have a slower rate of progression, but this observation represented a trend, not a statistically significant finding. They noted, as had others before them, the fundamental difference between the respective cohort survival curves of PD and postencephalitic parkinsonism (PEP). That is, patients with PEP were often severely disabled, but the majority tended to reach a stable plateau early in the course and to show little sign of deterioration even after 20 or more years of symptoms.

Progression of PD occurs early in the majority of cases. Figure 7.1 illustrates this phenomenon among 70 patients in the Hoehn and Yahr series during the first 4 years. The variability of the decline in neurological function is evident as is the rapidity of deterioration in the 37% of patients who reached Stages 3 and 4 (Stage 1 is mild disability and Stage 4 is severe disability on the Hoehn and Yahr scale). These proportions were in close agreement with the findings of Schwab and of Mjones. Twenty to 30% of patients from all three series were still classified as mildly impaired (Stages 1 and 2) 10 years after onset of disease.

Shortly after its introduction in 1967, levodopa radically changed the face of PD. The great majority of patients were transformed from disabled to independent within a few weeks or months of their beginning treatment. The excellent response aroused speculation that levodopa was a cure for PD, but the reality of progressive disease quickly dispelled this early optimism. Experience showed clearly that levodopa responders demonstrated the same unpredictable tendency to become disabled with time that was known before the drug's introduction [6,44]. Moreover, unusual adverse effects of treatment were observed. Cotzias et al. [16] described early choreiform involuntary movements and wearing-off effect in responders whose baseline was advanced disease. Barbeau [4] observed a syndrome in chronic drug users that was characterized by progressing motor impairment, involuntary movements and mental confusion. By the middle 1970's it was becoming clear that levopoda offered effective symptomatic relief to the majority of users, but that it did not substantially change the natural history of the disease in the long run for a given patient. Progression of disability was the rule for most patients, irrespective of the severity of symptoms at the start of treatment and the degree of early responses [84].

The spectrum of levodopa's undesirable effects has gradually been extending as new observations enter the literature each year. Moreover, the combined impact of levodopa and the older anticholinergic drugs has further increased the complexity of managing PD. The goal of this chapter is to review the complications and controversies surrounding the use of drugs in PD within the context of the advanced stages of the disease. The use and problems associated with the newer dopamine agonists (bromocriptine and pergolide) are discussed thoroughly in Chapters 3 and 6.

PROBLEMS OF ADVANCED PARKINSON'S DISEASE

Increasing Motor and Postural Disability

Postural instability is the great nemesis of patients with advancing disease. It causes the intractable difficulties of gait (freezing, festination, falling, hesitation), and because treatment of these is ultimately ineffective, the appearance of progressive postural instability marks a major turning point in outlook for doctor and patient alike. Except for the fortunate persons whose disease follows a benign course (especially those who remain in Stage 1), most patients will eventually confront the problems related to loss of postural control. The typical disturbance of gait usually begins with shortening of the stride or transient hesitation of the first few steps immediately after getting out of a chair. It is a self-correcting nuisance at first, but with the passage of time the tendency is for the feet to stick ever more tenaciously to the floor, often gluing the patient to the spot until another person comes along to assist with the unsticking. Doorways become a major obstacle; parkinsonian feet will almost predictably freeze at the threshold of a room, except at those embarrassing times in the doctor's office, when the patient comes to demonstrate the frustrating problem and walks smoothly inspite of himself. Eventually, hesitation and freezing become so dominant that walking is difficult anywhere and everywhere. Family members usually learn to perform "tricks" that will assist the patient's locomotion. A foot placed immediately in front of the stalled patient at a right angle to the direction of movement is a surprisingly effective way to restart forward motion. Stepping up stairs, stepping through the rungs of an imaginary, horizontally placed ladder, or over low objects regularly spaced in the patient's path, or marching to a cadence are usually much better executed than is ordinary walking. One patient, a musician, found that the regular beat of a tabletop metronome paced his walking at home, and a portable postauricular metronome provided a helpful cadence when he was outside. There is no ready explanation for why these simple maneuvers work, just as there is no clear understanding of the mechanisms underlying the basic symptom. As the tendency to freeze becomes more prominent, tricks become less effective, and many patients are forced to give up unassisted walking, resigning themselves to "furniture" walking at home and assisted walking otuside.

The threat of falling due to loss of postural-righting reflexes is a source of even greater disability than hesitation or freezing. Many patients become terrified of walking even before the appearance of obvious difficulty, because of the growing perception that simply being on one's feet is precarious. The occurrence of the first unwarned fall is usually a memorable event. Shoulder, rib, hip, and skull contusions or fractures are frequent enough to aggravate an already worsening predicament for those who ignore the need for a change in walking behavior. Rotator-cuff injuries often lead to pain and to permanent weakness of abduction of the proximal arm. The combination of proximal weakness and deteriorating dexterity of the hands attributable to PD can render an upper extremity completely useless. Hip fractures and head injuries are potentially lethal consequences of careless, unassisted walking. Each can lead to prolonged hospitalization and accelerated disabilty. It is usually difficult to convince a patient to give up walking, but in obviously dangerous circumstances an assertive physician must insist that all precautionary measures be implemented to prevent injury.

Speech
Impairment of speech, the basic instrument of human communication, is almost universal in PD. Loss of speech amplification is the most com-

mon defect. There is no reserve capacity for raising one's voice. Talking on the telephone becomes especially intimidating, because the muffling effect of the machine compounds the communication barrier. In early disease, parkinsonian hypophonia is usually mild and easily compensated, although many self-conscious patients perceive the speech problem to be more troublesome than it actually is. As the symptom worsens, speech tends to become more unintelligible. Volume drops even lower, the tongue becomes sluggish, and words are slurred. Palilalia, the lingual equivalent of festinating steps, is the uncontrolled repetition of syllables, words, or phrases, which obstruct the natural flow of orderly syntax by essentially freezing speech. Palilalic speech was commonly seen during the era of PEP; it is not as common today because PEP has all but disappeared. Deteriorating speech often parallels progressive impairment of balance and gait. Speech, like handwriting or any repetitive movement (shaving, knocking on a door, etc.) may start boldly before losing amplitude and, by the end of a sentence, trailing off into a whisper. Poorly sustained contraction and rigidity of vocal cords is the most likely cause of this phenomenon.

Breathing

Ventilatory dysfunction is frequently overlooked in PD, but it can occur and, rarely, is life threatening. There are 2 principal defects in the apparatus of breathing in PD: chest-wall rigidity causing hypoventilation, and upper-airways obstruction secondary to hypertonic and incoordinated striated muscles in and around the vocal cords and larynx [81]. The latter is probably more significant, as suggested by the findings of a recent study by Vincken et al. that showed a surprisingly high prevalence of resistance to expiratory outflow in patients with advanced PD [81]. Abnormalities of the diaphragm and chest wall were thought to be negligible. The amount of upper-airway resistance correlated directly with the degree of overall parkinsonian severity in these patients, thus, supporting a notion that the rigidity of upper-airway musculature parallels rigidity throughout the body in PD. Bannister et al. documented the high frequency of upper-airway obstruction in patients with the Shy-Drager form of multiple system atrophy [3]. They found gross and histologic evidence of neurogenic atrophy of crisoarytenoid muscles in 3 postmortem cases, but no convincing loss of neurons in either the nucleus ambiguus or of axons in the efferent nerve supply to muscle. The cause of the atrophy is unknown, although disuse imposed by rigidity is most likely.

It is probable that the disturbances in phonation, swallowing, and breathing associated with advanced disease are caused by a progressive increase in tone of the numerous sets of striated muscles that surround the upper airway and pharynx. Therefore, as parkinsonism becomes more debilitating, patients tend to develop severe hypophonia, dysphagia, aspiration pneumonia, laryngeal stridor, and even ventilatory failure if vocal cord paralysis supervenes [63]. Vincken et al. found the measurement of forced expiratory flow in liters/minute (FEVI) to be a simple test to screen for potential ventilatory problems in parkinsonian patients who have respiratory symptoms [81].

Swallowing

The majority of parkinsonians have little trouble swallowing solid food or liquid until late in the course of the disease. Akinesia of swallowing is the probable reason for drooling (sialorrhea), because production of saliva is normal in PD [61]. Drooling is usually confined to the period of sleep in early disease if it occurs at all. Later, it is an embarrassing daytime phenomenon, frequently reduced by the antiakinesic effect of levodopa or the drying effect of anticholinergics. As with other problems in severely disabled patients, drooling may eventually become totally unresponsive to all drugs.

Symptomatic dysphagia occurs in the setting of advanced disease and tends to reflect the severity of the patient's generalized motor impairment. At times, swallowing function can be relatively spared in the face of severe, global akinesia—as seen during drug holiday—or, conversely, it can be disproportionately bad when other motor symptoms are mild. Achalasia of the proximal esophagus was the underlying mechanism favored by some experts to explain the dysphagia of PD [62], but others have noted that esophageal dysfunction is much more often due to a more generalized incoordiantion of swallowing, affecting the tongue, pharynx, and upper esophagus [42]. Rare patients may, in fact, be helped by cricopharyngeal myotomy (surgical sectioning of unrelaxed cricopharyngeal muscles). However, this simple procedure may be technically successful but provide little or no improvement in swallowing; selection of the best candidate for this operation is, therefore, imprecise. It should be done only after a careful radiographic evaluation shows a characteristic pattern of sustained contraction of cricopharyngeal muscles in the pattern or achalasia.

Sex

Libido tends to be an early casualty as PD progresses, although there is no organic basis for the loss of sexual drive. Impotence in men is probably common and is certainly underreported. In a survey by Longstreth et al. [43], patients ranked sex and handwriting as the 2 most important losses in advanced disease, in addition to the more familiar problems of precarious walking, fatigue, and loss of independence. Shortly after its introduction, levodopa gained brief notoriety as an aphrodisiac, but experience proved that patients who responded dramatically to the motor effect were sexually charged because of unleashed normal urges, not because of any specific pharmacological action of the drug. As the disease advances, sex drive diminishes, but antidepressants or sex therapy in some cases help to reverse the decline in function. Antiparkinsonian drugs usually have little impact on sex drive, except that occasional patients (mostly men) or their spouses will report hyperactive sexual urges in late stages of the disease. Dopaminergic drugs may be culpable [11]. If persistent, the behavior becomes more nuisance than pleasure to an elderly female spouse.

Anticholinergics can be indirectly involved with the loss of sexual drive. Many elderly men with PD have had latent prostatism activated by innocent use of low doses of trihexyphenidyl (Artane), benztropin (Cogentin), and other drugs from this group, leading to cystoscopy, prostatectomy, and, occasionally, impotence as an adverse effect of prostate surgery. These synthetic atropinics should be used cautiously and in low dosage to prevent prostatic, mental, and pulmonic complications of well-intentioned treatment.

Bladder

Frequency and urgency of urination become increasingly troublesome as the parkinsonian syndrome advances. Early in the evolution of bladder dysfunction, cystometric measurement of the pressure-volume relationship will usually disclose a reduction in filling capacity, with an early, urgent need to void due to uncontrolled contractions of the detrusor muscle. These are the classic findings of an uninhibited bladder due to loss of descending corticospinal and autonomic inputs typically seen in advancing stages of PD. Later in the course of the disease, the small-capacity uninhibited bladder may become flaccid and hypotonic, especially in patients whose parkinsonian syndrome has other features of autonomic insufficiency (e.g., Shy-Drager). Recurrent cystitis and prolonged use of antiparkinson drugs can injure the bladder's detrusor muscle sufficiently to account for this change in some patients. Urinary urgency is replaced by loss of bladder sensation and overflow incontinence, but increased frequency of urination may not be affected.

Men with PD may have the added problem of age-related obstructive uropathy secondary to prostatic enlargement. Prostatic hypertrophy and its symptoms of frequency, urgency, and nocturia can mimic the uninhibited bladder or can add to the trouble already caused by disinhibition. It is not uncommon for a patient to have symptoms of prostatism, loss of inhibition, and infected bladder at the same time. The components of such a compound problem can only be dissected by careful urologic assessment, usually employing cystoscopy, cystometrics, and urinary culture. Uninhibited contractions can sometimes be relieved by propantheline, a smooth muscle antispasmodic, which is less likely to cross the blood-brain barrier than hyoscine and other members of this group and, therefore, less likely to cause mental confusion. Cholinomimetics, like Urecholine, and timed voiding may help the hypotonic bladder, but most patients with a flaccid detrusor will eventually need intermittent catheterization, either by a family member or visiting nurse.

Gastrointestinal System

Motility in the GI tract is slowed by aging, but not additionally by PD [22]. However, parkinsonian patients are plagued by constipation, usually for a combination of reasons, including inactivity and use of antiparkinson drugs. A few studies [2] have suggested that the sympathetic innervation of the GI tract is abnormal in PD, but if such a defect does occur, it is probably minor, except in the Shy-Drager syndrome.

Slowed motility of the GI tract, especially the stomach, is critical to the mobilization of drugs in PD. Because of delayed emptying time, drugs may stay too long in the stomach and not move onto the proximal duodenum, where transport into the bloodstream occurs. Levodopa held too long in the stomach may be converted there by gastric dopa decarboxylase to dopamine, which cannot cross the blood-brain barrier. Anticholinergic agents slow motility even more [2] and, therefore, can be counterproductive when added to levodopa in the clinic to achieve additional antiparkinsonian effect. As a practical matter, the mixing of dopaminergics and anticholinergics is well tolerated by most patients. Anticholinergics should probably be avoided in very old patients, not only because of age-related loss of gastric motility, but also because of the heightened risk of mental confusion and urinary retention due to latent obstructive uropathy.

Cognitive Changes

Chapter 9 reviews this subject in detail, but a brief discussion is included here because of its importance as a cause of severe disability in advanced disease. Dementia appears to be more than a random component of the parkinsonian syndrome and is the focus of active debate for a number of reasons [76]. Publications on its nature and prevalence over the last 50 years have reflected a broad spectrum of opinion, in part because of varying research methodologies applied to the collection of data. In many studies the criteria for diagnosis of dementia are inadequate and the confounding effect of antiparkinson drugs has not been properly considered. Moreover, nondementing cognitive and affective disorders appear to be so commonly associated with PD that they have aroused additional, separate controversy. There is some evidence to suggest that the dementia of PD is merely coexisting Alzheimer's Disease—2 common diseases with overlapping borders affecting a susceptible, aging population [67]. Current information on the subject is not complete enough to permit a definitive conclusion about the exact pathophysiology of parkinsonian dementia [31].

Aside from the debate over nomenclature and causal mechanisms, the neurologist wants to know how commonly dementia and cognitive disorders occur in PD and what kind of effect these problems will have on treatment. The best estimate of the prevalence of dementia, using the criteria of *DSM III,* is 20% [12]. Other cognitive syndromes occur (mnestic, mild confusional, paranoid thinking, etc.), but frequency is hard to estimate for these lesser conditions that fail to meet criteria for dementia. Our own experience suggests that frank dementia can be diagnosed in 10-15%, while another 10-15% will have the "other" cognitive problems (inattention, forgetfulness) that definitely interfere with normal intellectual function, but either do not worsen or remain isolated without further evolution. Most investigators have found advancing age and declining motor functions to be the most important risk factors for mental deterioration in PD [54]. Drugs, especially the anticholinergics, always have the potential for making mental function worse (it is worth noting that of all the antiparkinsonism drugs Sinemet probably has the safest therapeutic margin for mental side effects). As PD advances, mental and motor functions often deteriorate in lockstep, creating a major dilemma for the treating physician, especially when confusion and visual hallucinations signal the appearance of drug intoxication. The doctor must choose either to maintain the amount of antiparkinsonian medication necessary to preserve mobility at the expense of mentation, or, conversely, to reduce medication to improve mentation at the expense of mobility. This Hobson's choice is always difficult, but most patients and families will choose the latter option.

PROBLEMS ASSOCIATED WITH ANTIPARKINSONIAN MEDICATIONS

Levodopa in its current combined formulation with carbidopa (Sinemet) has become the cornerstone of effective pharmacotherapy in PD, despite the multitude of complications that have been attributed to its use in the 20 years since it was introduced. All other drugs are less potent, although experience with the dopamine agonists (especially bromocriptine and pergolide) indicates that these agents are effective as monotherapy in early PD [49,80] but not for advanced states, when dopamine agonists work best in conjunction with Sinemet. Anticholinergics have been used to treat PD for almost 100 years. Now, as then, they are modestly effective in early disease for suppression of tremor and relief of rigidity. Occasional patients will report a salutary effect on the speed of movement, often demonstrated by the deterioration that occurs upon withdrawal of the drug when it appears to have lost its efficacy. The therapeutic margin is narrower with the anticholinergics than with any of the other antiparkinsonism drugs. The adverse effects are usually hard to tolerate because the relatively small benefit often fails to compensate for the offensiveness of the side effects. In the final analysis, the most exciting challenge to the treating physician is the possibility that each drug can be manipulated skillfully—singly or in combination—to achieve maximal benefit for stage of disease with least adverse reaction.

Anticholinergics

Atropine was the first agent used to treat the tremor and rigidity of PD in the late 1800s. A succession of synthetic agents appeared in the early to middle 20th century, and until the advent of levodopa in 1967, the range of medical therapy for PD consisted almost entirely of the various members of this drug family. Amantadine was not introduced as antiparkinsonian therapy until 1969 [73]. It has been estimated that the average improvement in overall neurologic function in patients taking anticholinergic drugs is 20%, compared with the 50% to 75% attributable to levodopa [38]. These agents usually suppress tremor, rigidity (and associated muscle pain), but have a smaller effect on bradykinesia, gait, balance, and postural instability. The specific drugs covered by the anticholinergic heading that are currently in the U.S. pharmacopia include:

1. Trihexiphenidyl (Artane)
2. Benztropin (Cogentin)
3. Procyclidine (Kemadrin)
4. Cycrimine (Pagitane)

For convenience of discussion, I am also including the antihistamines diphenhydramine (Benadryl), ethopropazine (Parsidol), and orphenadrine (Disipal); each has a variable anticholinergic effect with a smaller tendency to cause adverse reactions.

Mental Side Effects

Disruption of recent memory and the ability to form new memories is a common, circumscribed complaint among users of anticholinergics [71]. Loss of memory is also observed as part of the global confusional state that occurs with a high frequency among elderly parkinsonians; visual hallucinations may be a component of this symptom complex. Patients with advancing motor problems and preexisting cognitive abnormalities have the highest risk of mental decompensation when anticholinergics are used. A common setting for this sort of trouble is illustrated by the following hypothetical case history:

> Patient X takes Sinemet but the parkinsonian symptoms are inadequately controlled despite maximal dosing. The doctor decides that a second drug is a rational adjunctive step and starts an anticholinergic at a "reasonable" dosage. However, X has recently begun to develop progressive loss of intellectual abilities that have been subtle enough to escape the physician's notice; the added drug burden is immediately overwhelming and X rapidly becomes confused and agitated; visual hallucinations are pronounced.

In retrospect there were 2 errors in judgment: First, the use of an anticholinergic drug in a patient with emerging cognitive loss is probably contraindicated; at best the risk:benefit ratio is high, and use of the drug will most probably be transitory. Cognitive dysfunction and dementia in PD may be caused in part by degeneration of acetylcholine-producing cells in the nucleus basalis of Meynert, the same region implicated in the pathogenesis of Alzheimer's disease [83]. Antagonism of an already-failing cholinergic system will theoretically aggravate the cognitive functions that correlate with cholinergic activity (e.g., memory) and cause acute, clinically obvious worsening of the previously unobtrusive mental impairment.

Second, the "reasonable" starting dose may have been too high. It is always prudent to initiate any antiparkinsonian drug with the smallest possible amount, and gradually increment to the level at which a significant positive or negative response occurs. Pharmcological gradualism may prevent side effects altogether, or at least permit early detection of potentially serious adverse reactions. This practice takes time and a willingness to endure the uncertainty of outcome, but it is an indispensible strategem when using drugs to manage PD.

Urinary Retention and the Prostate

Perhaps the second most important risk of anticholinergic drug therapy is urinary retention in men due to aggravation of underlying obstructive uropathy. The possibility of prostatic hypertrophy must always be considered before anticholinergic treatment is initiated. Most neurologists who treat patients with PD eventually consult a urologist, and it is appropriate to ask for help promptly if urinary function becomes problematic. Many patients will actually require urologic evaluation before anticholinergic treatment, if careful history discloses the familiar symptoms that could lead to major trouble after starting medication.

Withdrawal Reactions

Anticholinergics can be effective, but the typical clinical response tends to be incomplete. Many patients will decide to continue the drugs if the net effect is substantially positive. Others will perceive that any benefit they are receiving is not worth the price they are forced to pay in side effects. Still others will have no qualms about stopping medication, because the response has been totally negative or inconsequential. Withdrawal of any antiparkinsonian drugs, *especially the anticholinergics,* should *never* be done abruptly, except under the urgent demand of acute intoxication. Rapid withdrawal can cause all symptoms to become significantly worse within 24 hours, probably because of the disruption of a central pharmacological equilibrium associated with prolonged blockade of acetylcholine neurons, independent of the underlying chemical pathophysiology of the disease. Fortunately, this type of deterioration is spontaneously reversible, but it may take days or in some cases weeks for an affected patient to recover the previous baseline. The following case illustrates the point:

MB is a 70-year-old man with a 6-month history of shuffling gait. Trihexiphenidyl (Artane) was started at the time of the diagnosis of PD, and he improved on a dose of 1 mg, 3 times a day. However, after several months he began to notice dry mouth and forgetfulness. The neurologic examination showed moderate parkinsonism (stooped posture, hypophonic speech, festinating gait, mild postural instability, but no tremor) and mild impairment of recent memory. Artane was stopped in preparation for starting Sinemet. There was no change in status for 3 days, except for improved memory, but on the 4th day he began to feel much slower, and he gradually lost the ability to get out of a chair, turn in bed, or dress independently. Urinary frequency increased dramatically. He also had pains in all joints and muscles, and was so anxious that he was short of breath and could not sleep. Sinemet was started 6 days after onset of the deterioration (10-100, 3 times daily) without effect, and Artane was resumed at the prior dose. By the 13th day he had improved on the combination of Sinemet and Artane, although his wife noticed intermittent, mild confusion. Motor function gradually returned to the prewithdrawal baseline, but mental function did not return to normal until Artane was *slowly* withdrawn 6 months later.

Withdrawal of an anticholinergic should be extended over 7 to 10 days in order to avoid this type of reaction. If symptoms worsen as the drug is being tapered, returning to a slightly higher dose can stabilize the patient's condition; withdrawal can be resumed or aborted if the reemergence of parkinsonian symptoms at the end of the 7 to 10 days indicates that the drug is actually providing a more lasting benefit than either doctor or patient had appreciated.

Comparative Efficacy

Despite the narrow therapeutic margin of all anticholinergic and antihistaminic drugs, some members of this pharmaceutical subgroup are better tolerated than others. Most patients will find that a positive or negative response to a given drug usually predicts the same response to others in the same category. Nevertheless, it is often useful to try 1 or even 2 additional anticholinergic/antihistaminics in succession (e.g., trihexiphenidyl, followed by diphenhydramine, then benztropin) if the first trial is unsuccessful, especially if the reason for failure is the appearance of side effects at subtherapeutic dosage levels. Severe adverse reaction to low doses of an anticholinergic, however, would predict poor tolerance for all other drugs in the group. Multiple trials would be inappropriate in such a patient, who probably has an underlying cognitive disorder.

Levodopa

The success of levodopa as replacement therapy for a deficient neurotransmitter in PD was, in retrospect, the fulfillment of an impossible dream. Although the road to market was circuitous and difficult, it only took 8 years between Ehringer and Hornykiewicz' discovery that dopamine was depleted in the parkinsonian brain [21] and the dramatic demonstration by Cotzias that an oral form of levodopa could reverse many of the symptoms of PD in the living patient [15]. During those years of experimentation, dopa (dihydroxyphenylalanine) was tested in its D and D,L racemic forms and found to be either ineffective or poorly tolerated. Finally, by the middle 1960s, Cotzias had removed the last major obstacle to convenient clinical use by showing that slow induction and incrementation of the L-form (levodopa) could prevent severe dose-limiting nausea and vomiting. The earliest randomized clinical trials confirmed the anecdotal impressions that levodopa was a dramatic breakthrough in the treatment to PD. Moreover, its development represented a compelling model for the eventual treatment of other degenerative neuronopathies of the central nervous system that secondarily deplete specific neurotransmitters. Levodopa has stood the test of time. It remains, after 20 years, the reference standard for pharmacotherapy in neurology. Unfortunately, no other degenerative neurologic disease has yet followed the same favorable story line.

The elegant simplicity of the idea of levodopa initially seemed too good to be true. Many initially believed that levodopa replacement was a cure for PD, but this halcyon view was rapidly eclipsed by the lengthening shadow of empirical proof showing continued progression of all signs of the disease despite maximal therapy [6,30,74,79]. By the middle 1970s virtually all investigators of PD in the levodopa era were convinced that the progressive nature of PD had not been substantially altered, although quality of life and age-adjusted mortality rates were favorably affected [19,33,46]. Moreover, the emergence of a host of new and unanticipated problems associated with long-term treatment began to create fears among the experts that levodopa, for all its wondrous benefits, might be ultimately harmful [4]. The simplicity of the idea of replacement therapy, thus, ran afoul of the practical complexity of the interactions between the drug and its disease. Figure 7.2 is a pictorial representation of these overlapping domains (disease versus drug) and the specific clinical problems that are reviewed and discussed below. The order of listing starts with problems encountered early in treatment (e.g., nausea) and advances to those encountered later (e.g., motor fluctuations).

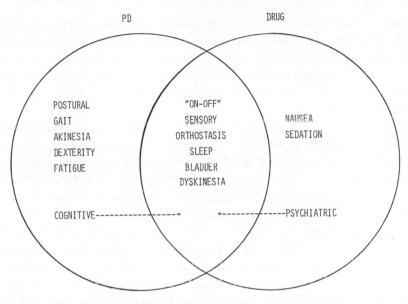

Figure 7.2 Problems in progressive PD, attributable to PD, antiparkinsonian drugs, and their interaction, are represented within the two overlapping circles.

Gastrointestinal Side Effects

Users of levodopa had nausea and vomiting so frequently that many potentially responsive patients were unable to tolerate a high-enough dose to derive benefit. The presumed cause of the problem had nothing to do with the GI tract, but rather was related to the emetic action of high plasma levels of dopamine at the area postrema, the vomiting center, which lies just under the floor of the fourth ventricle in the medulla and is one of the few regions of the brain that lies outside of and is not protected by the blood-brain barrier (BBB). Nausea was a significant barrier to effective treatment because each patient required a large amount of levodopa to overpower the short-circuiting effect of peripheral dopa decarboxylase, which converts 99% of oral levodopa to dopamine systemically and renders it impermeable to the BBB. High plasma dopamine levels trigger nausea and vomiting, as well as pronounced sympathomimetic clinical signs such as tachycardia, elevated blood pressure, pupillary dilatation, lid retraction, and tremulousness. Bartholini and Pletscher [7] were the first to suggest that the peripheral conversion of dopa to dopamine could be suppressed by pharmacological inhibition of dopa decarboxylase. They postulated that, as a result of such intervention, the amount of ingested levodopa necessary for a central effect could be greatly reduced, thereby preventing the number and severity of adverse systemic effects attributed to large quantities of peripherally converted dopamine. Clinical trials showed that carbidopa, the decarboxylase inhibitor, when combined with levodopa, permitted an 80% reduction in effective levodopa dosage; as well, it eliminated nausea and vomiting in the majority of users.

A single tablet containing a 10 to 1 ratio of levodopa to carbidopa was marketed as Sinemet (Merck) in 1975, and as a result levodopa usage was immediately extended to a significant new group of parkinsonians previously unable to tolerate the drug. In 1980 a 4:1 levodopa:carbidopa formulation was introduced (Sinemet 25-100) to make inhibition of dopa decarboxylase even more complete (total saturation of the peripheral enzyme appears to occur at 75 mg to 80 mg per day). Sinemet, except in rare instances, has replaced levodopa alone as the first line of dopaminergic treatment. Nausea is still a problem for some, but mainly during the first stage of treatment before patients adjust to medication; even then, it rarely interferes with adequate dosing. Slow induction, ingestion with meals or snacks, substitution of Sinemet 25-100 for 10-100, and crushing pills are effective techniques for overcoming nausea. These same techniques usually become unnecessary later, when many patients discover that the potency of Sinemet is enhanced if it is ingested on an empty stomach, because of the tendency for simultaneously ingested protein in food to impede the duodenal absorption and plasma transport of levodopa [57]. In the relatively few patients for whom Sinemet causes intolerable nausea at any dose, there are several other options: Carbidopa without levodopa has been formulated as a separate agent (Lodosyn-Merck) for use with Sinemet. Some patients may require more carbidopa than the 80 mg per day that theorectically saturates the enzyme (dopa decarboxylase) substrate. Drugs that block the emetic action of dopamine at the area postrema have also been helpful to those relatively few patients who develop nausea on very small doses of Sinemet. Domperidone is one such agent that has been successful, because it selectively blocks dopamine receptors in the area postrema and is excluded from other parts of the brain (and striatal dopamine receptors) by the BBB [1]. Metoclopramide (Reglan), a dopamine antagonist with a similar mode or action, also combats nausea and vomiting, but because it crosses the BBB, it has the tendency to worsen parkinsonism by blocking medullary and striatal dopamine receptors. Domepridone has had mixed results in clinical trials, but in our experience at the Graduate Hospital Movement Disorder

Center, it has enabled 8 of 12 patients with previously intractable nausea to achieve a therapeutic response to Sinemet, bromocriptine, or pergolide for the first time. Domerpidone is an experimental drug available on request from Janssen Pharmaceuticals.

Dyskinesias/Abnormal Involuntary Movements (AIMS)

Levodopa's propensity to produce undesirable adventitious movements was noted early in its history. Cotzias [16] observed that some of his most severely impaired patients showed peak-dose choreoathetosis of the arms, legs, head and neck concurrently with clinical improvement shortly after initiating treatment. Such dyskinesias have become a familiar signature of chronic levodopa usage. Patients often perceive the movements as an index of drug efficacy, titrating dosage to a level that strikes a balance between dsykinesias and optimal functional mobility. This middle zone of good function is relatively simple to find and sustain early in the disease. With increasing duration of disease, however, AIMS become more complicated. The movements tend to become more pronounced on the same or smaller doses of Sinemet—the clinical equivalent of denervation supersensitivity of striatal dopamine receptors—and more difficult to modulate by means of fine tuning through changes in Sinemet dosages. Most patients who use Sinemet eventually develop a fluctuating response (the wearing-off reaction), which, when mixed with increasingly complicated AIMS, causes an inexorable loss of the desirable middle region of the dose-response curve (see below for further discussion).

Levodopa-induced dystonia was also recognized early as a complication of treatment. The profile of dystonia, however, was more convoluted than peak-dose choreoathetosis, which tends to occur in one narrow phase of the plasma kinetic cycle when improvement is maximal. Dystonia is different: It can parallel, precede, follow, or disassociate from improvement and is often painful [68].

Myoclonus is the third dopa-related AIM that will be included here. It commonly occurs around or during sleep, but may also be a component of the chaotic cluster of AIMS that characterize advanced disease and the fluctuating response.

Choreoathetosis

Choreoathetoid movements are the most common of the AIMS associated with chronic levodopa therapy. Patients whose first symptoms of PD began before the age of 50 are unusually prone to early dyskinesias

[29], although the majority of levodopa users at any age will report or demonstrate writhing, jerky, usually low-amplitude, nonstereotyped AIMS, recognizable as chorea, athetosis or (most commonly) a blend of the 2 at anytime if the dose of the drug is high enough. The bodily distribution of movement is variable, but any and all parts can be affected, from blinking eyes to restless toes. Some patients develop wild, failing movements on minute doses of Sinemet—as small as 25 to 50 mg. Others can tolerate large amounts of drug with little or no excessive movement. This variability is not surprising in a disease that is all but defined by variability, but the mechanism, presumably related in some way to differential receptor sensitivity/density, is unknown but explorable with new techniques, such as Positron Emission Tomography (PET).

Chorea does not occur among the rare persons who take levodopa because of a mistaken diagnosis of PD. Thus, chorea in users of levodopa tends to confirm the diagnosis of Lewy body PD, and is a clinical indicator that striatal dopamine receptors are: 1) not impaired by degeneration of the nigrostriatal pathway; and 2) supersensitive to dopamine's impact as a transmitter. This supersensitivity presumably derives from nigrostriatal denervation and is most convincingly demonstrated in human and experimental (6-hydroxydopamine) hemiparkinsonism, when ipsilateral choreiform AIMS or contraversive turning occur, respectively, in response to receptor stimulation by levodopa or dopamine agonists [65].

Choreoathetosis is so common among parkinsonians using Sinemet that it probably has little value as a predictor of any of the possible types of future drug responsiveness [30], including sustained response, fluctuations, or progressive loss of efficacy.

Dystonia
Dystonic postures of the hands and feet are basic to the pathophysiology of untreated PD [25]. The *striatal hand* is almost pathognomonic and is a reliable sign in differentiating PD from other neurologic disorders that affect voluntary movement. At times PD overlaps primary dystonia (torsion dystonia) in a single patient or family (Parkinson-dystonia complex) [59], thereby revealing the closely intertwined pathophysiologic mechanisms that produce the 2 clinical syndromes. Although dystonia can be a manifestation of dopamine deficiency in untreated PD, it is a common and disabling complication of chronic levodopa therapy, usually occurring at the peak of levodopa's clinical effect, but also during the "off" period after the clinical effect has dissipated, or on arising in the morning

after a night without the drug [50]. Patients typically describe the posturing as twisting, stiffening, or tightening of the affected part(s), commonly the limbs on the more parkinsonian side, and especially the foot. Dystonia can be unilateral or generalized, involving the limbs, face and axial muscles.

Dystonia is distinct from chorea in several ways. First, as clinical phenomena the two have different kinetic characteristics: Chorea is writhing, hypotonic, and fluid; agonists and antagonists are equally active. Dystonia, on the other hand, is restrictive and hypertonic; either flexors or extensors (not both) tend to dominate, and a static, twisted posture is the rule, although superimposed sudden, jerking movement is a frequent accompaniment. Second, whereas chorea is usually a peak-dose effect, dystonia occurs in various parts of the dosage cycle. This is a major therapeutic point, because the adjustments required to relieve chorea or dystonia may not only be different but must also reflect an understanding of levodopa's pharmacokinetics. Chorea and dystonia occurring as a peak-dose effect can be abolished by reducing the Sinemet dose; "off" dystonia must be treated by increasing the dosage (see below under Fluctuations for further discussion). Early morning dystonia of the foot, also an off dystonic rection, resolves after ingestion of the first Sinemet dose of the day. Third, the intense muscular contractions of dystonia tend to be painful, occasionally requiring strong analgesics for relief. Sustained periods of dystonia can be associated with spontaneous breakdown of muscle fibers (rhabdomyolysis), elevation of creatine phosphokinase (CPK) in the blood, fever, and, in rare instances, acute renal failure secondary to deposition of myoglobin in renal tubules.

Some patients have a combination of chorea and dystonia; the familiar pattern and borders of each tends to be blurred in the admixture. An observed, videotaped single-dose tolerance test is a useful technique for dissecting the various components of the more complex levodopa-induced AIMS (see below under Fluctuations).

Myoclonus

A sudden, moderate-amplitude jerking movement of segments of the body with quick relaxation is a reasonsable definition of myoclonus. It is often bilaterally expressed in the same narrow range of body segments (as with both arms or legs), and can have a startlingly abrupt onset. Myoclonus is usually not a feature of untreated PD, although it has been reported [36]. The most common setting for myoclonus is sleep and its temporal surround. Patients taking Sinemet may notice sudden jerking of their legs as sleep is near, or be awakened by the movements during sleep. The movements subside if Sinemet dosage is reduced. The compicated response to Sinemet that is associated with years of usage may include a lightninglike, myoclonic component in addition to chorea and dystonia.

Psychiatric and Cognitive Problems

Confusional states and pure visual hallucinosis (usually in the form of nonthreatening, sedentary, unfamiliar people in the immediate environment) are the two most common problems encountered during the course of chronic, sustained pharmacological treatment of PD (see Chapter 9 for more discussion). Many patients with otherwise normal mental function can hallucinate on surprisingly small amounts of anticholinergic or dopaminergic drugs. Others tolerate large amounts of these drugs without showing the slightest sign of mental clouding.

The variability of such drug reactions is typical of most other aspects of PD; it also supports the general impression that drug-induced hallucinations and acute confusional episodes do not predict the later cognitive deterioration that tends to occur in advanced disease in approximately 20% of parkinsonians [12,23]. Paranoid delusions and auditory hallucinations are uncommon, usually developing more gradually than other mental syndromes in patients who are required to use large doses of antiparkinsonian drugs for progressive motor deterioration. Resolution of the more complicated psychiatric symptoms can take days or weeks after all offending medications have been withdrawn. Unfortunately, the long-term cost of treating an acute or subacute mental crisis under these circumstances is usually a significant reduction in motor function, dictated by the necessity of a permanent decrease in dosage of otherwise therapeutically effective antiparkinsonian drugs. The following case history illustrates the problem:

DD is a 54-year-old woman with a 10-year history of slowly progressive parkinsonism that began with rest tremor and rigidity of the right arm. As the symptoms and signs became increasingly generalized and disabling, she required larger doses of dopaminergic drugs to prevent an acceleration of motor deterioration. She had responded well for several years to Sinemet, to Sinemet and bromocriptine (Parlodel) when Sinemet alone failed, and to Sinemet and pergolide mesylate after Sinemet and bromocriptine began to lose efficacy. She was admitted to the hospital in mid-1986 because of the emergence of a severely disruptive mental syndrome, characterized by intense visual hallucinations, paranoid delusions that the people she hallucinated were plotting to harm her, uncontrollable crying, and agitation. Daily medications at that time included 1000 mg of Sinemet (25-100) in 10 divided doses, and 15 mg of pergolide in 5 divided doses. Neuropsychiatric exam on admission showed that she was alert, oriented, agitated, frightened, tearful, and was actively hallucinating. Parkinsonian rigidity, akinesia, hypophonic speech, shuffling giat and postural instability were moderately severe. Doses of both antiparkinsonian drugs were reduced (mainly the pergolide), and after 6 weeks of a trial-and-error search for the right combination of medications (including two episodes of severe akinesia with dystonic posturing immediately after small doses of thioridazine and of trifluperazine, respectively), an acceptable balance between positive and negative effects of Sinemet and pergolide was found: The patient was discharged with a clear sensorium, but was forced to tolerate more tremor and much less mobility than before hospitalization.

There are rare patients who have visual hallucinations in a drug-free state, possibly as an unusual feature of an evolving parkinsonian dementia.

Postural Hypotension

Severe postural hypotension is a rare complication of Sinemet therapy, but a mild drop in blood pressure on standing is a common cause of postural light-headedness and occasional syncope. Like many of the problems associated with Sinemet use, postural hypotension tends to occur in advanced states of the disease, often in conjunction with fluctuations or progressive loss of the drug's efficacy. Autonomic insufficiency is basic to the pathology of PD, because sympathetic neurons in the intermediolateral cell column of the thoracic spinal cord are variably affected during the course of the disease. The minor significance of autonomic insufficiency in the clinical spectrum of PD is a marker that distinctly separates PD from the Shy-Drager or the striatonigral variant of multisystem neuronal atrophy (MSA), although some patients present with or evolve symptoms and signs that overlap the two entities. A severely hypotensive response to a small dose of Sinemet or other dopaminergic medication in an otherwise typical parkinsonian should suggest the diagnosis of MSA rather than PD.

Postural hypotension, when severe, can be a dose-limiting barrier to the optimal use of Sinemet. Various pharmacologic and physical remedies have been proposed [9,10,18] but the most effective (if not the easiest) treatment is the prudent use of the mineralocorticoid 9-alpha, fludrocortisone (Florinef). The starting dose is 0.1 mg once or twice a day, supplemented by dietary salt. Florinef works through 2 mechanisms: First, its earliest but temporary effect is to expand intravascular (plasma) volume by promoting reabsorption of sodium from the proximal tubule of the kidney. Second, and more importantly, it increases vascular peripheral resistance by enhancing the vasoconstrictive effect of circulating norepinepherine [17]. Florinef has little hypertensive effect if the patient is salt depleted, and is potentially dangerous to use in patients with borderline or overtly failing cardiac function. Doses above approximately 0.4 mg are counterproductive because sodium retention and peripheral vasoconstriction are already maximal at that dosage level. Higher doses merely cause a linear increase in potassium loss, which occurs as a result of Florinef's impact on ion exchange at the proximal renal tubule (one molecule of sodium retained for one molecule of potassium expended).

It is important to emphasize the need for salt supplementation in the majority of patients. If dietary salt is not sufficient to maintain blood pressure in an adequate range, salt tablets (1 g sodium chloride per tablet) can be prescribed to titrate blood pressure against salt intake. Elevation of the head of the patient's bed during sleep is also an important feature of management, because recumbency can promote sodium loss through enhanced renal perfusion. Adverse consequences of chronic use of Florinef include pedal edema, congestive heart failure, hypokalemic metabolic alkalosis, and supine hypertension. Each can be avoided with careful management (support hose, low dosage, potassium supplements, etc.) but supine hypertension is probably the most common [14], and it can be difficult to control. It is also easily overlooked, because blood pressure is commonly measured only in the seated and standing positions in the doctor's office. The patient's principal caretaker should be taught to check blood pressure at home in all positions, so that significant supine elevations can be detected. Reduction of salt intake or Florinef itself may be required to treat the problem; elevating the head of the bed can be effective. Some brittle patients may absolutely need hypertensive doses of florinef and/or salt to permit even minimal standing and walking. Hydralazine (Apresoline) in low dosage (40-100 mg per day), or selected beta-blockers, have the potential for lowering supine blood pressure without affecting standing blood pressure, and will help the occasional patient [9,10].

Sensory Complaints

A variety of subjective sensations are frequently reported by chronic Sinemet users, such as facial flushing, feelings of intense heat, paresthesias, pain, and sweating. Most of these are intermittent but the degree of discomfort can be substantial. Flushing and heat tend to occur at peak-dose times. The face often turns red transiently; clothing may feel too constricting and the skin overly sensitive, as if burned. Sweating tends to occur in paroxysmal waves, drenching clothes, pajamas, nightgowns, or bedsheets. Although not greatly disabling, frequent sweats are an extreme nuisance. Paresthesias usually affect the legs in the evening when the patient is tired and ready to relax or go to bed. The sensation has been likened to insects crawling under the skin, annoying pinpricks, and the like. There is usually an associated need to walk, an action that seems to suppress the abnormal sensation. Akathisia, a term meaning "not to sit," might best describe the restlessness that can only be relieved by shifting the affected parts in chair or bed, or by walking. A rare patient will notice severe paresthesias as a dose of Sinemet is wearing off. The next dose will relieve the symptom, but it recurs regularly during "off" periods. Off-period sensory phenomena, like off-dystonia, have the potential for converting a usually akinetic or passive phase of the response cycle into a harrowing mixture of passive and actively unpleasant components. One such patient under my care was ultimately unable to tolerate Sinemet at all because of the intensity of the off-paresthesias, which gradually subsided after Sinemet was completely withdrawn. Without Sinemet she progressed to severe Stage IV dependency, but preferred this condition to the "terrible" feelings she was forced to endure every 2 hours during the day while taking Sinemet.

Pain is frequently a vexing problem in PD [68]. It can distract from early recognition of the correct underlying cause and delay diagnosis. Pain is a familiar companion to levodopa-induced peak-dose or off-dystonia, and in another setting it may accompany several cogwheel rigidity and subside when tone is relaxed by a favorable drug response. Thus, antiparkinsonian drugs can cause or relieve pain, or have no impact at all. It is notable how often pain masquerades as a symptom of distress in other organ systems, leading to an unproductive search for an underlying cause. Yet parkin-

sonians do develop other illnesses, which may present as painful disturbances.

The mechanisms underlying these peculiar problems can only be surmised. Flushing, sensations of heat, and sweating may result from the catecholamine effect of dopa peripherally converted to dopamine. An unstable sympathetic nervous system related to the advancing pathology of
PD could somehow be responsible. Acetylcholine can also be implicated.
However, there is virtually no evidence to support a particular pathophysiology. Sweating was commonly observed in PD long before levodopa was
introduced, especially among postencephalitics. Various drugs have been
tried to control the entire array of sensory complaints, but none has been
effective enough to favor any single pharmacologic hypothesis.

Problems of Sleep and Arousal

Levodopa has a central alerting action in experimental animals, and it
can cause a similar response in humans as well—as adrenergic effects such
as lid retraction, anxiety, sweating, tachycardia, and premature cardiac
contractions [13]. To most parkinsonians, sleep restores motor function,
even late in the disease. The best time of day for many is the first hour
after awakening, even if the most recent dose of antiparkinsonian medicaiton was taken 8 hours before at bedtime. During this time, the typical
patient can get up, shave, bathe, and dress with little or no assistance.
Sleep benefit tends to be most pronounced early on, and is less impressive as disability increases, especially when fluctuations start to appear.
Yet, even in advanced disease when self-care is greatly compromised and
there is ample reason to despair about the loss of freedom, some patients
will be consoled by the preservation of that morning hour of independence and wonder why it cannot be extended to the rest of their day.

Levodopa's classic alerting effect is often unknown to patients with PD,
who may feel uplifted during the honeymoon phase of first exposure to
the drug, but who are commonly sedated after each dose later in the
course of their disease. This type of reaction is often a prelude to reversal of the sleep cycle: somnolence or napping all day and restless wake-
fulness at night. The elderly patient with mental confusion or frank
dementia is the usual victim. Dextroamphetamine (Dexedrine) or methyl-
phenidate (Ritalin) may help to restore order to the sleep cycle, but the
benefit is usually transient. Nevertheless, either drug taken in a small dose
once or twice a day is worth a trial in selected patients.

Table 7.1 Levodopa Response and Prognostic Subgroups in Parkinsonism

A. Good prognosis:
    Sustained Response to L-dopa and/or slow progression
B. Guarded or Poor Prognosis:
    Changing response to L-dopa and/or rapid progression
    1. Primary drug failure:
        Never responders (PSP, SND, OPCA)
    2. Secondary drug failure:
        a. With and without fluctuations
        b. With and without cognitive impairment

PSP = progressive supranuclear palsey; SND = striatonigral degeneration;
OPCA = livoponto-cerebellar atrophy

Most of the antiparkinsonian medications can cause active dreaming. Few patients are truly disturbed by this effect, although spouses or caretakers are often startled or awakened by the noisy dreamer. It is rare for a drug to be discontinued for this reason.

The Prognosis of Parkinson's disease and the Response to Levodopa

The quality of the typical patient's favorable response to Sinemet tends to change with increasing duration of use. The levodopa honeymoon lasts for 6 to 12 months in most responders. During this period, dosing is 2, 3 or 4 times daily, usually with meals and at bedtime; benefit is usually sustained throughout day and night. With the passage of time this long-duration response (LDR) gives way in the majority to one of two patterns: 1) fluctuations, dominated by the wearing-off or short-duration response (SDR); or 2) progressive loss of drug efficacy without significant fluctuations [40]. Patients in either of these subgroups have manifest signs of increasing disability, but for mysterious reasons the clinical features of the implied progression of underlying disease diverge into more or less distinct directions. A minority of parkinsonians will maintain a good and lasting response to Sinemet. Many of these will have Stage I disease that does not spread. Others have a tremor-dominant syndrome that lacks the more disabling and pernicious components of advanced disease, such as postural instability, mental incompetence, and severe generalized akinesia. These relatively few patients have truly benign disease.

Table 7.1 represents an arbitrary attempt to divide the universe of treated PD into three prognostic subgroups. The division is purely empirical and, therefore, may ultimately be invalidated by future clarification of the pathophysiology of progressive PD. Fluctuations and progressive loss of drug efficacy are the focus of the discussion that follows.

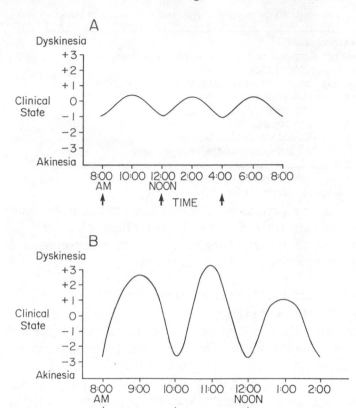

Figure 7.3 (A). Mildly fluctuating response to oral levodopa occurring early in the evolution of progressive parkinsonism, but usually after several years of levodopa usage. Time of dosing is indicated by arrows on the baseline. (B). Widely fluctuating response to levodopa, marked by prominent swings between severe akinesia and pronounced dyskinesia, as seen in advanced disease and as a further evolution from the mild fluctuations of Figure 7.3A.

Fluctuations

Overview and Pathophysiology

The wearing-off response (end-of-dose deterioration) usually appears for the first time several years after initially successful treatment [40]. The majority of all Sinemet users eventually fluctuate [44,30], particularly young parkinsonians at any stage and patients at any age with advanced disease at initiation of treatment with Sinemet. The change can be noticeable in some cases within weeks of starting treatment [16,37]. The earliest experience is a mild, but distinct feeling of activated movement (the "on" response) 15 to 30 minutes after ingestion of a dose, lasting 3 to 4 hours before it gradually fades into the bradykinetic "off" phase of the drug's response curve (see Figure 7.3a). The rise and fall of the "on" and "off" responses may remain stable, or the degree of fluctuation may become more pronounced and the duration of the "on" response shorter until it parallels the 90-minute plasma half-life of levodopa (Figure 7.3b). The treating physician and patient together discover that the interdose interval must be shortened eventually from 4, to 3, to 2 hourly, as dictated by the patient's perceived need to avoid deep troughs in an undulating dose-response curve.

The underlying mechanism invoked by many experts to explain the emerging dominance of the SDR in chronic Sinemet users is the progressive death of nigral neurons and a corresponding decline in the capacity of the remaining nigrostriatal neurons to take up exogenous dopa, convert it to dopamine, then store the dopamine in vesicles and tonically release it from the presynaptic axonal terminals across the striatal synapse to activate postsynaptic dopamine receptors. In health, the nigrostriatal dopamine pathway is the site of smooth execution of all these functions, which in the aggregate help produce normal voluntary movement. When the first signs of parkinsonism appear, an estimated 80% of nigrostriatal dopamine has already been depleted by the insidious nigral pathology of PD [8]. It is assumed that the surviving nigral neurons are numerically adequate to handle exogenous dopa and modulate its pharmacologic effects; hence, the smooth response to Sinemet in early PD. Progressive degeneration of the last 20% of nigral neurons not only undermines modulation, but also depletes the nigral stores of the converting enzyme dopa decarboxylase (DD). Because a therapeutic response depends on effective conversion, it must take place in the brain outside the nigral system as these neurons become severely depopulated. Melamed et al. [51] have shown that alternate conversion probably takes place in small neurons of the caudate and putamen. Other neighboring sites of conversion are likely, because DD is ubiquitous in the brain. Thus, a controlled and well-modulated system of delivering dopamine to its striatal receptors withers in parallel with the progressive nigrostriatal degeneration of PD. This growing void is filled by a system of bolus transport of orally ingested dopa into the brain, where striatal dopamine receptors are activated by a relatively unmodulated shower of transmitter, fluctuating in delayed synchrony with the 90-minute plasma half-life of levodopa.

Perhaps the most impressive feature of the fluctuating response to Sinemet, even years after it first begins to surface, is the degree to which post synaptic dopamine receptors seem to retain their responsiveness to exogenous transmitter despite severe loss of the presynaptic nigrostriatal pathway. Aside from the possibility that postsynaptic striatal dopamine receptors increase as a result of denervation supersensitivity, dopamine receptors appear not to be affected by the natural pathophysiology of PD. This does not take into account the potential for "down regulation" of dopamine receptors by chronic exposure to exogenous levodopa [39,69,70]. Therefore, the smooth response of the first use of levodopa might be regained if Sinemet's short half-life could be circumvented by a delivery system that could release the drug at a constant, highly controllable rate—through the skin, subcutaneous fat, or directly into the blood. Experimental trials employing each of these routes are currently underway [60,66,77].

It is important to note that the changing pattern of the response to levodopa from LDR to SDR appears not to be derived from plasma pharmacokinetics, which remain the same irrespective of duration of illness or treatment, and age of the patient [58]. In other words, the change must be attributed to intracerebral factors rather than to the way the drug is handled between duodenal uptake and transport to the brain. Spencer and Wooten have shown in rats with unilateral lesions (6-hydroxydopamine) of the nigrostriatal pathway that striatal dopamine peaks at a lower level and declines faster on the lesioned side versus contralateral control following the parenteral administration of levodopa [75]. They infer from these experimental data that intracerebral levodopa kinetics are similarly altered in human PD, attributable mainly to the disruption of transmitter delivery associated with the loss of presynaptic storage sites.

Clinical Characteristics

The onset of the SDR is usually difficult to pinpoint. Early on, patients will notice a subtle lift 15 to 30 minutes after taking a dose of Sinemet and a gradual decline in speed of movement 3 or 4 hours later (see Figure 7.3a). If dyskinesias accompany the peak-dose effect, they tend to be mild; nigrostriatal storage is probably adequate to keep the range of the excursion from "on" to "off" within reasonable bounds, preventing a large dyskinetic overshoot in the motor response. At this point, shortening the interval between Sinemet doses will usually limit the amount of motor slowing during the off period. Once the patient adjusts the dosage and learns to accept SDR as a new phase in the natural evolution of the Sinemet-PD relationship, the actual level of disability is only slightly greater than before, depending upon social and occuaptional demands. There are numerous instances, however, wherein the appearance of fluctuations causes enough additional disability to force some highly skilled workers (usually young parkinsonians) to leave their jobs or take early retirement.

SDR may remain stable and manageable for an indefinite period, or the swings from "on" to "off" may become more extreme, even chaotic, with prominent and troublesome dyskinesias characterizing the "on" response and total immobility characterizing the "off." Most patients find that the Sinemet interdose interval will eventually need to be shortened in time to 2 hours, although the time frame for making the change and the prospect for a satisfactory resolution are unpredictable and variable, like everything else in PD. The following case illustrates how the wearing-off reaction typically evolves:

> TS first noticed rest tremor of the left arm in 1980 at the age of 62, and it was attributed to anxiety. A shuffling, unsteady gait developed 6 months later, but the diagnosis of PD was not made until walking became more difficult, a full year after the tremor first appeared. Sinemet gave excellent relief at a dose of 10-100 3 times daily for about a year, but the tremor and disturbance of gait gradually reappeared. She began to notice mild fluctuations and peak-dose choreiform dyskinesias in early 1983, requiring a gradual increase in Sinemet dosage over the next 9 months to 25-250, 5 times per day (every 3 hours from 9 AM to 9 PM). Fluctuations continued to be mild, although the period of good response gradually shortened to 2 hours, and postural instability became more incapacitating. She fell frequently despite careful self-monitoring; on one occasion she dislocated the left shoulder and developed permanent weakness in the muscles of the rotator cuff. She needed a walker but could not manipulate it because of the newly weakened left arm. The addition of bromocriptine to Sinemet caused severe nausea at a low dosage and was discontinued after a few days. Amantadine suppressed the tremor and temporarily improved the gait for several months, but she began to require human support when she walked and noticed wider swings in the response to Sinemet, the dosage of which was maintained at the same level. Dyskinesias were moderately severe at peak dose and were a mixture of choreiform involuntary movements and dystonic postures, moreso on the left. The "off" periods were increasingly akinetic. In mid-1986 she noticed an accelerated increase in the severity of the dyskinesias over a period of several weeks and was admitted urgently to hospital for treatment of

"seizures" affecting the entire body, but more on the left side. The "seizures" were treated with phenytoin briefly until it became clear that the involuntary movements were induced by Sinemet and were not epileptic. Sinemet dosage was reduced gradually to 25-100, 4 times a day and the dyskinesias subsided, although the akinesia of all movement that followed made her more dependent in all activities of daily living. An attempt to increase the dosage of Sinemet by an additional 150 mg was defeated by the immediate reappearance of severe dyskinesias.

This patient has a familiar story as victim of the shrinking middle; that is, the progressive loss of the middle region of the response curve that represents a well-modulated balance between excessive (dyskinetic) and insufficient (akinetic) mobility. Nutt and coworkers [58] analyzed this phenomenon and found that the threshold of minimal responsiveness (average plasma dopa level of 8-10 nmol/mL) in patients with advanced disease and fluctuations was all or nothing: Above the critical level, patients had a positive motor response but with uncontrollable dyskinesias; below it, they could barely move. This intractable clinical state, in which there is a rapid decline in tolerance for previously effective doses of oral Sinemet, presumably correlates with the severe loss of storage capacity decribed above. The end result in many cases is an irreversible advance in the staging of the disease to a permanent Hoehn and Yahr stage IV or V.

Fluctuations eventually conform with the pattern described in the case of TS in the majority of patients. Early on, the kinetic response to Sinemet is proportionate to the height of the blood dopa level. There is a recognizable sequence of: 1) parkinsonism; 2) initial *I*mprovement; 3) peak-dose effect (with or without *D*yskinesias); 4) post-peak *I*mprovement; 5) "wearing-off" and return of parkinsonism. This has been called the IDI (improvement, dyskinesia, improvement) response pattern by Meunter et al. [55,56]. Later, the all-or-none response (see above) tends to prevail. Approximately 10% of fluctuators will demonstrate a reversal of the IDI sequence (Meunter's DID or dyskinesia-improvement-dyskinesia response) as well as the relationship between plasma dopa levels and clinical response as follows: 1) parkinsonism; 2) a brief episode of *D*yskinesia (often dystonia), occurring shortly after ingestion of the day's first dose of Sinemet; 3) *I*mprovement as the plasma dopa level moves toward its peak; 4) more prolonged *D*yskinesia at the end of the cycle as plasma (and brain) dopa levels slowly drift back to baseline; and 5) the "off" clinical state [5,41,55]. Figure 7.4 shows that IDI and DID have opposing ther-

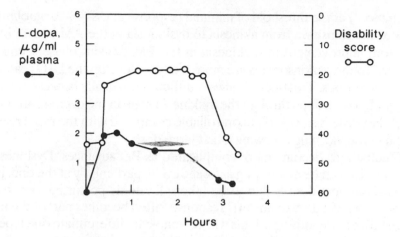

Figure 7.4A. The IDI response to a single dose of 200 mg of levodopa. The change in the disability score roughly parallels the plasma levodopa curve; dyskinesias occur near plasma peak, preceded and followed by improvement. The disability score ranges from 0 (normal) to 60 (severe). From Meunter et al., 1977, reprinted by permission.

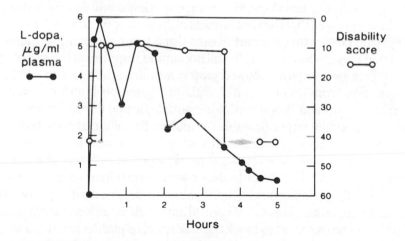

Figure 7.4B. The DID response to levodopa. Biphasic dyskinesias occur before and after improvement in a patient following a 1500 mg dose of levodopa, ingested at time 0. From Meunter et al., 1977, reprinted by permission

apeutic implications. In the case of IDI (and patient TS above), the dose of Sinemet will need to be titrated to balance dyskinesias against immobility. In the case of DID, the dyskinesia is abolished by increasing the dosage of Sinemet to raise plasma dopa above the narrowly critical zone (commonly at the threshold of minimal responsiveness—8-10 nmol/mL), where the transition from akinesia to dyskinesia in the AM boost phase or from improvement to dyskinesia in the PM descent phase seems to occur. Young parkinsonians are more likely to develop the DID reaction than older ones. Treatment is always difficult, especially because the descent of plasma dopa through the dyskinesia zone in the evening after the day's last dose is slow and uncontrollable compared with the rapid rise of dopa in the morning following a first large dose.

Fluctuations become more complicated as PD advances. Dyskinesias can coexist with tremor during a dosage cycle, particularly at the end, just before the next dose is due to be taken. Dystonic posturing, occurring either as a peak dose or an "off" response, often becomes part of the mix. Some otherwise astute patients will be unable to differentiate one type of involuntary movement from another in the confusing tangle and will adjust medication in the wrong direction as they try to correct the imbalance.

The "true on-off" reaction is a variant of the wearing-off phenomenon that was first described as a separate clinicopharmacologic entity because of the apparent randomness of the clinical oscillations in relation to the dosing schedule of levodopa. However, experience and careful investigation have revealed that the randomness of "true on-off" is probably caused by specific factors that prevent plasma dopa from exceeding a threshold level that corresponds with a clinical dopamine response at the site of striatal dopamine receptors: Slowed gastric motility, stress and anxiety, and competition from dietary amino acids are common interfering factors [52,57,58]. Nutt and Woodward, for example, found during levodopa-infusion studies that unpredicatable or random fluctuations occurred when steady-state plasma concentrations of levodopa hovered around the threshold for minimum-effective clinical response (4-8 nmol/mL). Concentrations above 10 nmol/mL always gave a sustained response. Drug-resistant "off" periods often occur if Sinemet is ingested with or soon after a meal, because the transport of neutral amino acids derived from ingested protein can be expected to block the transport of plasma levodopa across the BBB. Quinn and Marsden have shown that a *dose-related* wearing-off pattern can be uncovered in patients with complicated fluctuations if the response cycles are analyzed cumulatively over a period of several days [66]. Likewise, Obesso [60] has successfully smoothed seemingly random fluctuations in patients treated with subcutaneous lisuride, a water-soluble ergot-derived direct dopamine agonist. In the final analysis, the "true on-off" reaction probably does not exist, except in rare patients with fluctuations that cannot be attributed to the vagaries of plasma kinetics

or environmental circumstances. The current state of knowledge, therefore, supports the hypothesis that the fluctuating response "largely reflects the action of a short-lived drug with erratic absorption and distribution in patients critically dependent upon delivery of levodopa to the striatum for normal motor function, and is not the result of a novel or idiosyncratic response to levodopa" [58].

The problematic patient may need to spend a few hours or even a day
in the doctor's office under direct, uninterrupted observation so that an
accurate temporal profile of the dose-response pattern can be generated.
Careful observation of the patient's unfolding response to the day's first
dose of Sinemet may be a crucial step in resolving any uncertainty surrounding the nature and timing of the motor fluctuations. The information usually helps to determine what to do next with what medication. Ex-
ceptional patients whose fluctuations are too complicated or disabling for
outpatient resolution will require hospitalization for several days or more
for intensive scrutiny and readjustment of the program of treatment.

Progressive Loss of Drug Efficacy without Fluctuations

Patients covered under this descriptive heading usually show an initial
good response to Sinemet for an unpredictable length of time, following
which a steady decline in neurologic function (often with mental impairment) eclipses the prior favorable response. In the worst case, motor and
mental functions deteriorate in parallel, forcing a retreat from aggressive
drug therapy because of the inevitable poor tolerance for all medications
(e.g., the case of DD above). These patients lose still more motor function as a result of the reduced dosages of antiparkinsonian drugs and tend
to follow a steady decline to severe dependency. Unlike the fluctuators,
who maintain their essential drug responsiveness despite the loss of modulation, patients with progressive loss may have underlying striatal
pathology that disables postsynaptic dopamine receptors as a result of primary or transsynaptic degeneration [48], or a drug-induced down-regula-
tion of receptor function [32,69]. Moreover, the frequent coupling of progressive motor and mental symptoms suggests that a dopamine/acetylcho-
line deficiency state may be playing a unique role in the natural history of
patients in this subgroup [76].

Risks of Hospitalization

Most treatment options in PD can be exercised outside the hospital,
but some patients may require hospitalization if the following specific indications arise:

1. Newly diagnosed PD with severe disability that threatens to cause medical complications (such as pneumonia, phlebitis, etc.). Aggressive treatment in hospital (drugs and physical therapy) will telescope treatment time and prevent serious problems.
2. Severe intoxication by antiparkinsonian drugs.
3. Failure to control severe fluctuations with the best outpatient program.
4. Rapidly progressive symptoms in the face of maximal drug treatment.
5. Drug holiday.

Hospitalization should be undertaken only after careful advanced planning, because of the strong possibility that any program of inpatient management will be subverted by Murphy's Law. Despite best intentions, patients often do not get their medications on time, or the doses are wrong because an order was mistakenly written or read. Patients fall and hurt themselves because they walk about improperly attended in an unfamiliar environment. Older patients may become confused and belligerent, especially after sundown. Nurses without proper training in the sophisticated management of PD will not be alert to the special problems and needs of parkinsonians. The fluctuating response to Sinemet, for example, is always difficult to comprehend: How can a patient be alternately independent and helpless in such a short space of time?

Anger, frustration, and suspicion on both sides become serious impediments to effective treatment. Rarely, unwitting patients are victims of neglect and verbal and/or physical abuse by uncaring hospital workers, who are unable or unwilling to provide the requisite comfort that is taken for granted at home. Finally, some people just seem to "do poorly" in hospital, even when everything is done correctly, possibly because of the psychological trauma of being away from home and family. Then there are those patients who require admission for other medical or surgical problems that temporarily overshadow and destabilize the finely tuned control of the parkinsonian machine. Quite simply, hospitalization can be a terrifying experience under the best of circumstances. However, it also can be used effectively for the indications above if all human procedural components of management are meticulously arranged to prevent disaster.

Drug Holiday

Sweet et al. [78] were the first to observe a transiently enhanced response to levodopa in parkinsonian patients after periods of complete drug withdrawal lasting as long as 10 days. Direnfeld [20], Weiner [82], Goetz [24], and Kaye [34] have reported their individual experiences with drug withdrawal or drug "holiday" (DH) as an effective technique for reversing drug-induced side effects and signs of progressive parkinsonism in selected patients. Approximately 50% of patients appeared to respond favorably for up to 6 months or longer, irrespective of duration or severity of disease and dosage, or duration of levodopa therapy. Responders not only had fewer drug-induced side effects after DH, but achieved a higher level of neurologic function on reduced amounts of levodopa, compared with pre-holiday dosage. Each of these investigators used as a pharmacologic rationale the hypothetical notion that hallucinosis, fluctuations, and signs of declining drug efficacy associated wth chronic levodopa therapy were somehow related to the drug's desensitizing or down-regulating effect on striatal dopamine receptors. A temporary suspension of this deleterious pharmacologic bombardment during DH would allow receptors to resensitize and respond more like normal, following the reintroduction of levodopa. The net result of the successful DH, according to its proponents, would be to turn back the clock and recapture the more favorable drug response of early disease.

Since the concept of DH was first proposed, experience with its application has aroused criticism by some that its resensitizing effect on receptors and overall clinical benefit are at best highly transitory and at worst nonexistent [47]. Moreover, the considerable risk of dangerous complications (aspiration pneumonia, deep vein phlebitis and pulmonary embolus, psychological shock) occurring during the severely akinetic nadir of DH does not justify its routine use [45]. Receptor studies in a few human parkinsonian brains initially gave tentative support to the rationale of resensitization [39,70], but more recent evidence from a much larger sample contradicts the earlier work by showing no alteration of dopamine receptor density with respect to age, duration and severity of PD, or duration of levodopa therapy [27]. Finally, contrary to the popular notion that minimal dosing of levodopa protects against hypothetical long-term toxic effects of drug-related metabolites (especially superoxide free radicals), experience has shown that this sensible strategy offers no guarantee that progression or potentially drug-induced adverse effects will not occur [64]. Nevertheless, the single most compelling practical reason for continued application of the *idea* of a DH (perhaps not a complete or prolonged withdrawal of the drug) in some patients is the relief of increasingly uncontrollable dyskinesias and/or psychiatric side effects.

Drug holiday has been diversified to include weekend or single day or even single-dose withdrawals for treatment of patients with advanced disease and extreme response fluctuations who could not tolerate complete and prolonged cessation of levodopa therapy. Our own experience at the Graduate Hospital Movement Disorder Center has led us to abandon the complete DH in favor of a variety of the partial holiday techniques mentioned above. However, the DH story remains unfinished. Final answers pertaining to its true validity await the execution of appropriate clinical trials and studies using in vivo receptor-imaging techniques such as Positron Emission Tomography (PET) to elucidate quantitative and qualitative changes in receptor function during and after periods of drug withdrawal.

REFERENCES

1. Agid Y, Bonnet AM, Lhermitte F, et al: Bromocriptine associated with a peripheral dopamine blocking agent in treatment of Parkinson's disease. Lancet 1:570-572, 1979.
2. Algeri S, Cerletti C, Curcio M, et al: Effect of anticholinergic drugs on gastro-intestinal absorption of L-dopa in rats and man. Eur J Pharmacol 35:293-299, 1976.
3. Bannister R, Gibson W, Michaels L, Oppenheimer DR: Laryngeal abductor paralysis in multiple system atrophy. Brain 104:351-368, 1981.
4. Barbeau A: Long term side effects of levodopa. Lancet 1:395, 1971.
5. Barbeau A: Diphasic dyskinesia during levodopa therapy. Lancet 2:756, 1975.
6. Barbeau A: Six years of high-level levodopa therapy in severely akinetic parkinsonian patients. Arch Neurol 33:333-338, 1976.
7. Bartholini G, Pletscher A: Cerebral accumulation and metabolism of C14-dopa after selective inhibition of peripheral decarboxylase. J Pharmacol Exp Ther 161:14-20, 1968.
8. Bernheimer H, Birkmayer W, Hornykiewicz O, Jellinger K, Seitelberger R: Brain dopamine and the syndromes of Parkinson and Huntington. J Neuro Sci 20:415-455, 1973.
9. Blomquist CG: Orthostatic hypotension. Hypertension 8:722-731, 1986.
10. Bradshaw MJ, Edwards RTM: Postural hypotension: pathophysiology and management. Quart J Med 60:643-658, 1986.
11. Brown E, Brown GM, Kofman O, Quarrington B: Sexual function and affect in parkinsonian men treated with L-dopa. Am J Psych 135:1552-1555, 1978.
12. Brown RG, Marsden CD: How common is dementia in Parkinson's disease? Lancet 2:1262-1265, 1984.
13. Carlsson A: Basic concepts underlying recent developments in the field of Parkinson's disease. In McDowell FH, Marshall CH (eds): Recent Advances in Parkinson's Disease. FA Davis, pp 1-31, 1971.
14. Chobanian AV, Volicer L, Tifft CP, Gavras H, Liang CS, Faxon D: Minerolocorticoid-induced hypertension in patients with orthostatic hypotension. N Engl J Med 301:68-73, 1979.

15. Cotzias GC, VanWoert MH, Schiffer LM: Aromatic amino acids and modification of parkinsonism. N Engl J Med 276:374-379, 1967.
16. Cotzias GC, Papavasiliou PS, Gellene R: Modification of parkinsonism: chronic treatment with L-dopa. N Engl J Med 280:337-345, 1969.
17. Davies B, Bannister R, Sever P, Wilcox CS: The pressor action of noradrenaline, angiotensin and saralasin in chronic autonomic failure treated with fludrocortisone. Br J Clin Pharm 8:253-260, 1979.
18. Davies B, Bannister R, Sever RS: Indomethacin treatment of postural hypotension in autonomic failure. Br Med J 1:181, 1980.
19. Diamond SG, Markham GH: Present mortality in Parkinson's disease the ratio of observed to expected deaths with a method to calculate expected deaths. J Neurol Trans 38:259-269, 1976.
20. Direnfeld L, Spero L, Marotta J, Seeman P: The L-dopa on-off effect in Parkinson's disease: treatment by transient withdrawal and dopamine receptor resensitization. Ann Neurol 4:573-575, 1978.
21. Ehringer H, Hornykiewicz O: Verteilung von Noradrenalin und Dopamin (3-Hydroxytyramin) im Gehirn des Menschen und ihr Verhalten bei Erkrankungen des extrapyramidalen Systems. Klin Wschr 38:1236-1239, 1960.
22. Evans MA, Broe GA, Triggs EJ, et al: Gastric emptying rate and the systemic availability of levodopa in the elderly parkinsonian patient. Neurology 31:1288-1294, 1981.
23. Goetz CG, Tanner CM, Klawans HL: Pharmacology of hallucinations induced by long term drug therapy. Am J Psychiat 139:494-497, 1982.
24. Goetz CG, Tanner CM, Klawans HL: Drug holiday in the management of Parkinson disease. Clin Neuropharmacol 5:351-364, 1982.
25. Gortuai P: Deformities of hands and feet in parkinsonism and their reversibility by operation. J Neurol Neurosurg Psych 26:33-36, 1963.
26. Gowers WR: Paralysis agitans. In A Manual of Diseases of the Nervous System (American ed). Philadelphia, Blakiston, pp 995-1014, 1888.
27. Guttman M, Seeman P, Reynolds GP, et al: Dopamine D2 receptor density remains constant in treated Parkinson's disease. Ann Neurol 19:487-492, 1986.
28. Hoehn MM: Parkinsonism; onset, progression and mortality. Neurology (Minn) 17:427-442, 1967.
29. Hoehn MM: Parkinsonism treated with levodopa: progression and mortality. J Neurol Transm 19(suppl):253-264, 1983.
30. Hoehn MM: Parkinson's disease: progression and mortality. VIIIth International Symposium on Parkinson's disease, 1985.
31. Jellinger K: Pathology of parkinsonism. In Fahn S, Marsden D, Jenner P, Teychenne P (eds): Recent developments in Parkinson's disease. New York, Raven Press, pp 33-66, 1986.
32. Jenner P, Boyce S, Marsden CD: Effect of repeated L-dopa administration on striatal dopamine receptor function in the rat. In Fahn S, Marsden D, Jenner P, Teychenne P (eds): Recent Developments in Parkinson's Disease. New York, Raven Press, pp 189-203, 1986.
33. Joseph C, Chassan JB, Koch ML: Levodopa in Parkinson's disease. Ann Neurol 3:116-118, 1978.

34. Kaye JA, Feldman RG: Role of L-dopa holiday in the long term management of Parkinson's disease. Clin Neuropharm 9:1-13, 1986.

35. Klawans HL, Geotz C, Nauseida PA, Weiner WJ: Levodopa-induced dopamine receptor hypersensitivity. Ann Neurol 2:125-129, 1977.

36. Klawans HL, Tanner CM, McDermott TH: Myoclonus and Parkinson's disease. Clin Neuropharm 9:202-205, 1986.

37. Lang AE, Meadows JC, Parkes JD, Marsden CD: Early onset of the "on-off" phenomenon in children with symptomatic parkinsonism. J Neurol Neurosurg Psych 45:823-825, 1982.

38. Lang AE: Treatment of PD with agents other than levodopa and dopamine agonists: controversies and new approaches. Can J Neurol Sci 11:210-220, 1984.

39. Lee T, Seeman P, Rajput A, et al: Receptor basis for dopaminergic supersensitivity in Parkinson's disease. Nature 1273:59-61, 1978.

40. Lesser KP, Fahn S, Snider SR, et al: Analysis of the clinical problems in parkinsonism and the complications of long-term levodopa therapy. Neurology 29:1253-1260, 1979.

41. Lhermitte F, Agid Y, Signoret JC: Onset and end-of-dose levodopa- induced dyskinesias. Arch Neurol 35:261-263, 1978.

42. Logemann JA, Blonsky ER, Boshes B: Dysphagia in parkinsonism. JAMA 231:69-70, 1975.

43. Longstreth WT, Linde M: Sickness impact profile in Parkinson's disease. Neurology 34(suppl):207-208, 1984.

44. Marsden CD, Parkes JD: Success and problems of long-term levodopa therapy in Parkinson's disease. Lancet 1:345-349, 1977.

45. Marsden CD, Parkes JD, Quinn N: Fluctuations in disability in parkinson's disease-clinical aspects. In Marsden CD, Fahn S (eds): Movement Disorders. London, Butterworth, pp 96-122, 1981.

46. Martilla RJ, Rinne UK, Sartola T, Sonninen V: Mortality of patients with Parkinson's disease treated with levodopa. J Neurol 216:147-153, 1977.

47. Mayeux R, Stern Y, Mulvey K, Cote L: Reappraisal of temporary levodopa withdrawal ("drug holiday") in Parkinson's disease. N Engl J Med 313:724-728, 1985.

48. McNeill TH, Brown SA, Laphan TA, et al: Dendritic regression of medium spiny neurons of the striatum in Parkinson's disease. Neurology 36(suppl 1):74, 1986.

49. Mear JY, Barroche G, deSmet Y, et al: Pergolide in the treatment of Parkinson's disease. Neurology 34:983-986, 1984.

50. Melamed E: Early morning dystonia: A late side effect of long-term levodopa therapy in Parkinson's disease. Arch Neurol 36:308-310,1979.

51. Melamed E, Hefti F, Pettibone DJ, et al: Aromatic L-amino acid decarboxylase in rat corpus striatum: implications for action of L-dopa in parkinsonism. Neurology 31:651-655, 1978.

52. Melamed E, Bitton V, Zelig O: Delayed onset of responses to single doses of L-dopa in parkinsonian fluctuations on long-term L-dopa therapy. Clin Neuropharm 9:182-188, 1986.

53. Mjones H: Paralysis agitans: A clinical and genetic study. Acta Psychiatr Neurol Scand Suppl 54:1-195, 1949.

54. Mortimer JA, Pirozzolo RJ, Hansch EC, Webster DD: Relation of motor symptoms to intellectual deficits in Parkinson's disease. Neurology 32:133-137, 1982.

55. Muenter MD, Sharpless NS, Tyce GM, Darley FL: Patterns of dystonia ("I-D-I" and "D-I-D") in response to L-dopa therapy for Parkinson's disease. Mayo Clin Proc 52:163-174, 1977.

56. Muenter MD: Should levodopa therapy be started early or late? Can J Neurol Sci 11:195-199, 1984.

57. Nutt JG, Woodward WR, Hammestad JP, Carter JH, Anderson JL: The "on-off" phenomenon in Parkinson's disease: relation to levodopa absorption and transport. N Engl J Med 310:483-488, 1984.

58. Nutt JG, Woodward WR: Levodopa pharmacokinetics and pharmacodynamics in fluctuating parkinsonian patients. Neurology 36:739-744, 1986.

59. Nygaard TG, Duvoisin RC: Hereditary dystonia-parkinsonism syndrome of juvenile onset. Neurology 36:1424-1428, 1986.

60. Obeso JA, Martinez-Lage JM, Luguin MR: Lisuride infusion pump: a device for the treatment of motor fluctuations in Parkinson's disease. Lancet 1:467-470, 1986.

61. Pallis CA: Parkinsonism: Natural history and clinical features. Brit Med J 3:683-690, 1971.

62. Palmer ED: Dysphagia in parkinsonism. JAMA 229:1349, 1974.

63. Plasse HM, Lieberman AN: Bilateral vocal cord paralysis in Parkinson's disease. Arch Otolaryngol 107:252-253, 1981.

64. Poewe WH, Lees AJ, Stern GM: Low dose L-dopa therapy in Parkinson's disease: a 6-year followup study. Neurology 36:1528-1530, 1986.

65. Pycock CH, Marsden CD: Central dopaminergic receptor supersensitivity and its relevance to Parkinson's disease. J Neurol Sci 31:113-121, 1977.

66. Quinn NP, Parkes JD, Marsden CD: Control of on-off phenomenon by continuous IV infusion of levodopa. Neurology 34:1131-1136, 1984.

67. Quinn NP, Rossor MN, Marsden CD: Dementia and Parkinson's disease—Pathological and neurochemical consideration. Brit Med Bull 42:86-90, 1986.

68. Quinn NP, Lang AE, Koller WC, Marsden CD: Painful Parkinson's disease. Lancet 1:1366-1369, 1986.

69. Reches A, Wagner HR, Lewis VJ, et al: Chronic levodopa or pergolide administration induces down regulation of dopamine receptors in denervated striatum. Neurology 34:1208-1212, 1984.

70. Rinne UK, Lonnberg P, Koskinen V: Dopamine receptors in the parkinsonian brain. J Neural Transm 51:97-109, 1981.

71. Sadeh M, Braham J, Modan M: Effects of anticholinergic drugs on memory in PD. Arch Neurol 39:666-667, 1982.

72. Schwab RS: Progression and prognosis in Parkinson's disease. J Nerv Ment Dis 10:556, 1960.

73. Schwab RS, England AC, Poskanzer DC, Young RR: Amantadine in the treatment of Parkinson's disease. JAMA 208:1168-1170, 1969.

74. Shaw KM, Lees AJ, Stern GM: The impact of treatment with levodopa on Parkinson's disease. Quart J Med 49:283-293, 1980.

75. Spencer SE, Wooten GF: Altered pharmacokinetics of L-dopa metabolism in rat striatum deprived of dopaminergic innervation. Neurology 34:1105-1108, 1984.

76. Stern MB, Gur RC, Saykin AJ, Hurtig HI: Dementia of PD and AD: Is there a difference? J Am Geriat Soc 34:475-478, 1986.
77. Stoessl AJ, Clane DB, Maak E: (+)-4-propyl-9-hydroxynaphthoxazine (PHNO), a new dopamimetic, in treatment of parkinsonism. Lancet 2:1330-1331, 1985.
78. Sweet RD, Lee JE, Spiegel HE, McDowell FH: Enchanced response to low doses of levodopa after withdrawal from chronic treatment. Neurology 22:520-525, 1972.
79. Sweet RD, McDowell FH: Five years treatment of Parkinson's disease with levodopa: therapeutic results and survival of 100 patients. Ann Int Med 83:456-463, 1975.
80. Teychenne PF, Bergsrud D, Racej A, et al: Bromocriptine: low dose therapy in Parkinson's disease. Neurology 32:577-583, 1982.
81. Vincken WG, Gauthier SG. Involvement of upper-airway muscles in extrapyramidal disorders. N Engl J Med 311:438-442, 1984.
82. Weiner WJ, Perlik S, Koller WC, Nausieda PA, Klawans HL: The role of drug holiday in the management of Parkinson's disease. Neurology 30:1257-1261, 1980.
83. Whitehouse PJ, Price DL, Struble RG, Clark AW, Coyle JT, DeLong MR: Alzheimer's disease and senile dementia: loss of neurons in the basal forebrain. Science 215:1237-1239, 1982.
84. Yahr MD: Evaluation of long-term therapy in Parkinson's disease:mortality and therapeutic efficacy. In Birkmayer W, Hornykiewicz O, (eds): Advances in Parkinsonism. Basle: Editiones Roche, pp 444-455, 1976.

Chapter 8

Dopaminergic Agonists in the Treatment of Advanced Parkinson's Disease*

Christopher G. Goetz,
Caroline M. Tanner,
and Harold L. Klawans

THE CELLS THAT DIE AND ARE PRIMARILY RESPONSIBLE for the motor abnormalities of Parkinson's disease originate in the substantia nigra and project to the striatum. Striatal dopaminergic receptors become progressively denervated as the presynaptic degeneration progresses. Although levodopa, the precursor to dopamine itself, has traditionally been the major drug used to treat Parkinson's disease, in advanced cases, direct-acting dopaminergic agonists that stimulate striatal receptors offer at least four theoretical advantages over levodopa itself:

1. Levodopa has no pharmacologic effect on dopamine receptors; and its efficacy in Parkinson's disease depends on its conversion to dopamine by the enzyme dopa decarboxylase. As Parkinson's disease advances and the population of dopaminergic cells projecting to the striatum progressively declines, the activity of this enzyme also diminishes. Hence, in advanced Parkinson's disease, where less dopamine can be synthesized from administered levodopa, the use of an agent that bypasses the presynaptic area of dysfunction would theoretically be increasingly advantageous. Furthermore, the progressive decrease in dopa decarboxylase is not uniform in the brain but occurs predominantly in the nigrostriatal system. Therefore, in

* This work was supported by research funds from the Boothroyd Foundation and the United Parkinson Foundation, Chicago.

159

advanced Parkinson's disease, the converting enzyme is preferentially depleted in the area where it is needed, and the dose of levodopa required for this system may overactivate other dopaminergic systems in the brain and provoke adverse reactions. Agonists potentially can avoid this complication by acting independently of the synthetic dopaminergic enzyme system.

2. The half-life of levodopa is exceedingly short, and at least some of the motor fluctuations seen so frequently in advanced Parkinson's disease appear to relate to circulating levels of the drug; the agonists as a group have prolonged half-lives and therefore become the logical agents for patients with motor fluctuations related to wearing off of levodopa effect.

3. Levodopa modifies other neurotranmitter systems besides dopamine, including norepinephrine and serotonin. Agonists theoretically offer the advantage of specificity to the dopaminergic receptor populations in the central nervous system.

4. When levodopa is converted to dopamine, all dopaminergic receptor populations will be activated, not only those associated with the nigrostriatal dysfunction of Parkinson's disease, but also those of the hypothalamic prolactin circuit and the mesolimbic and mesocortical projections. Agonists offer the potential to activate selective dopaminergic receptor subgroups, and hence increase efficacy and avoid unwanted side effects related to indiscriminate dopaminergic stimulation.

Numerous dopaminergic agonists have been tested in the treatment of Parkinson's disease during the last 10 years, although only one, bromocriptine, is currently available in the United States. Several potent antiparkinsonian agents have been abandoned in the United States because of toxicity, including lergotrile, lisuride, mesulergine, and ciladopa. Liver toxicity and tumor production in animals were major toxic effects. This chapter reviews the clinical experience with the two ergot agents, bromocriptine, and pergolide (which is likely to be available to treating physicians in 1988 or 1989). The emphasis will be on practical recommendations for the use of these agents in advanced Parkinson's disease and the prevention and control of drug-induced toxicity.

In many of the published reports on agonists, patients with advanced disease have not been specifically separated from those with milder disabililty. For this summary, advanced disease is defined as a Hoehn and Yahr stage of III or greater—that is, the patient has specific postural reflex impairment at the time of agonist introduction and has been treated with levodopa chronically. Importantly, these patients not only have more marked Parkinson's disease than do milder cases, but they also often have significant toxic effects of chronic therapy, including motor fluctuations, hallucinations, confusion, sleep disturbance, and dyskinesia. Commonly they may also be significantly more demented than patients with mild Parkinson's disease, thereby enhancing their propensity to mental side effects from any centrally active drug. These issues all contribute to the challenge of safely introducing agonist therapy to this group of patients with advanced Parkinson's disease. Although both bromocriptine and pergolide have been used in early Parkinson's disease without levodopa, no large studies have been performed with agonist monotherapy in advanced Parkinson's disease patients. In most studies the agonists have simply been added to levodopa in an unblinded or blinded protocol, and patients' parkinsonism and toxic complications on levodopa/agonist combination were compared with levodopa alone. Clinical data on bromocriptine and pergolide will be discussed separately followed by comparative data on their relative safety and toxicity.

BROMOCRIPTINE

Efficacy

Bromocriptine was studied by Lieberman and colleagues [13] in 66 patients with advanced Parkinson's disease. At the time of the study, patients had increasing disability despite treatment with levodopa. Forty-five patients were able to tolerate at least 25 mg/daily of bromocriptine and the results of treatment were analyzed: Levodopa dose was reduced by 10% in the group and could be eliminated in 7 patients. Significant improvement occurred in the four cardinal features of Parkinson's disease—rigidity, tremor, bradykinesia and postural reflex impairment—as well as in overall disability. In 12 patients, follow-up data was obtained 1 year after bromocriptine introduction, and in 8 patients, bromocriptine remained effective. In a later publication [14], the same investigators reported that with time a progressive waning of efficacy developed with bromocriptine, although many patients remained improved or stable for at least 2 years. The mean dose of the first study was 45 mg/day, and 50 mg/day in the second group.

Other groups have demonstrated similar findings and documented not only global improvement but also fewer motor fluctuations and more frequent "on" time, where the patient is functional and relatively independent [1,4]. Kartzinel et al. [8] performed a double-blind study of bromocriptine and placebo as additions to levodopa therapy in 8 patients, and found overall improvement in the bromocriptine-levodopa group. Rigidity and tremor were better improved than was balance. Hoehn and Elton [5] studied patients with a wide variety of disabilities, and found that lower doses (maximal 20 mg/day) still improved motor function, although improvement was most significant in the milder cases. Only 2 of 6 patients at Stage IV improved more than 30%, whereas two thirds of patients at Stages II or III had more than 30% improvement.

Glantz et al. [2] investigated the effect of bromocriptine on random motor fluctuations unrelated to the time or dose of levodopa (true "on-off"). Twenty-three patients were studied prospectively, and 39% showed reduced "on-off," in that less immobility occurred and the frequency and unpredicatability of "off" episodes declined.

Almost all long-term studies have demonstrated that the beneficial effects of bromocriptine eventually wane. It is not clear whether this decline is due to progression of the Parkinson's disease itself or whether there is definite pharmacologic tolerance to the drug. Work in our medical center with drug holidays in patients who show progressive loss of efficacy to either levodopa or bromocriptine suggests that a 5-day drug-free period may resensitize the patient to antiparkinsonian drugs and will permit additional months of effective therapy. However, the hazards of severe immobilization that may occur during the holiday are not inconsequential (see Chapter 7).

Toxicity

Significant side effects, often necessitating discontinuation of bromocriptine in patients with advanced Parkinson's disease, have been reported in as high as 36% of patients [14]. With lower doses, only 15% of patients experienced side effects severe enough to require drug withdrawal [5]. Orthostatic hypotension is the most important side effect of bromocriptine in the early phase of drug introduction. Patients may become dizzy and even faint. In the various series reported above, orthostatic hypotension, lightheadedness, or syncope was detected in approximately 33% of patients. Usually, once the patient has received the drug for several doses, this effect wanes. Nausea and vomiting, presumably due at least in part to bromocriptine's direct stimulation of the dopaminergic receptors in the area postrema of the medulla can occur in 20-30% of patients and, unlike the nausea related to levodopa, will not be controlled with carbidopa. Domperidone, available in Europe and likely to become available in the United States, may offer a highly effective therapy for agonist-related nausea as well as levodopa-induced gastrointestinal complaints. Other less frequent complaints or complications include burning dysesthesias of the extremities that may relate to vasoconstrictive properties of ergot drugs, gastric hemorrhage, skin rash (livedo reticularis) of the lower legs, and rarely hepatitis or exacerbation of angina pectoris [5,13]. In the latter case, it is not clear whether the angina relates to vascular effects of the bromocriptine or whether the improved motor function of patients on bromocriptine permits their increased activity that now becomes limited by underlying cardiac dysfunction.

Neurologic and mental side effects are especially common in this group of advanced Parkinson's disease patients. Involuntary movements (dyskinesia), specifically chorea, increased in Lieberman's group as a whole, and in 40% in another study [1,13]. Besides chorea, peak-dose dystonia and myoclonus can occur with bromocriptine. Mental changes include agitation, confusion, depression, insomnia, nightmares, and hallucinations. These effects, occurring in 10-30% of patients, have been the most frequent cause of discontinuation of the drug [5]. The use of low-dose bromocriptine significantly decreased the prevalence of this side effect [5] (see Chapter 5). As a rule, it has been suggested that bromocriptine is associated with more psychiatric disturbance but less dyskinesia than levodopa [7].

Practical Recommendations

After 10 years of active work with bromocriptine, we have developed a number of guidelines that help us in the management of patients requiring agonist therapy. They reflect our method of care and should not be interpreted as absolute dicta. Patients with advanced Parkinson's disease who are receiving 2500 mg/day levodopa or Sinemet 60-600 and who are not adequately controlled are candidates for bromocriptine therapy. Poor control may be related to inadequate efficacy of levodopa, drug-induced side effects, or a combination of both. Patients who should not receive bromocriptine include those with a history of allergy to ergots, and those with severe cardiovascular disease or peptic ulceration. Because of significant mental side effects, bromocriptine must be used with extreme caution in patients with a history of hallucinations or dementia.

If bromocriptine is being introduced because the patient has a poor response to levodopa, no decrease in the levodopa dose is necessary. On the other hand, if bromocriptine is being used to improve efficacy and diminish levodopa-related side effects, the dose of levodopa should be decreased as the bromocriptine is increased. In our center, we usually start bromocriptine without decreasing levodopa during the first week. Because of its longer half-life, bromociptine probably does not reach steady-state plasma levels for several days. In the second week of therapy, as bromocriptine is increased, levodopa may be slightly deceased, usually by half tablets every 7-14 days. Our aim is to decrease the levodopa dose approximately 25%, avoid side effects, and prolong the duration of drug response and independent time for the patient.

Before bromocriptine is started, we measure the blood pressure with the patient supine, sitting and standing. If there is a systolic drop from one position to another of greater than 20 mm Hg, if the diastolic drops below 60, or if the patient is dizzy, we prefer to start the bromocriptine in the office. The patient will take the first dose and sit in an examining room for 4 hours. If he or she becomes dizzy or if further orthostatic drops occur when the blood pressure is measured each hour, a supine position is preferred. Only rarely is the hypotensive effect dramatic, but if it is, the patient may need to be hospitalized for the first several days of treatment.

If the blood pressure is stable before bromocriptine is introduced, we allow the patient to start the drug at home. Two options are available. For patients who do not get up at night, the first doses may be taken at bedtime in order to minimize the symptoms of any early hypotension. On the other hand, if the patient awakens frequently to urinate, the added effects of the bromocriptine on the natural hypotension induced by prolonged bed rest may be extremely hazardous; in such patients, we prefer that the patient start bromocriptine during the daytime, and we warn them to have a family member nearby and not to plan a strenuous or active schedule for that day.

The first dose of bromocriptine is usually 2.5 mg. If the patient complains of orthostatic symptoms, another trial dose should be given; if the dizziness is incapacitating, 1.25 mg/day can be tried for 3-5 days. In most cases, however, the patient will tolerate the first dose without symptoms. On the second day of therapy, we increase the total daily dose to 7.5, and aim to increase over two weeks to 10-15 mg/day. Evidence from clinical studies and animals has suggested that very low doses of agonists may activate presynaptic receptors and actually decrease dopaminergic activity at the postsynaptic receptors of the striatum. Very low doses of bromocriptine have even been used to treat choreic conditions including Huntington's disease and we have seen patients with advanced Parkinson's disease actually become more bradykinetic during the early phase of agonist therapy when they are receiving very low doses. Because of these concerns, we always try to treat the patient with at least 10 mg of bromocriptine daily, and to arrive at this moderate dose within 3 weeks of initiation of bromocriptine therapy. In our opinion, the controversies of low-dose versus high-dose bromocriptine seem more applicable to early phases of Parkinson's disease rather than to cases of advanced illness.

Once the dose of 10-15 mg/day is achieved, increases should be very slow, usually not more than 2.5 mg/day every 14 days. We have found that patients usually do not experience the therapeutic effects of bromocriptine fully until at least 5 days after an increase. This observation is of practical importance because physicians may be tempted to increase bromocriptine much more rapidly, and thereby overmedicate their patients unnecessarily; as Hoehn and Elton [5] demonstrated in their study of low-dose bromocriptine, toxicity is less common and less severe when the dose of bromocriptine is kept as low as possible.

Bromocriptine is an expensive drug, and for economic considerations, doses above 50 mg/day are uncommon. We have had experience with doses as high as 140 mg/day, and have been impressed that in patients who respond well at low doses without side effects, higher doses are increasingly effective. However, in patients who do not show significant improvement at 40 mg/day, we do not generally recommend further increases. Larsen et al. [10] found that the dose of bromocriptine needed to supress symptoms and signs of parkinsonism correlated well with the original disability and that patients with more advanced disease regularly required more than 30 mg/day. Although the duration of action of bromocriptine is several hours, the drug should be administered three, four, or more times daily in order to avoid high doses at each ingestion. We recommend that liver enzymes be checked yearly and that blood pressure be monitored regularly while a patient receives bromocriptine. Pleural thickening has also been reported occasionally with bromocriptine; an annual chest radiograph is also reasonable.

If toxic side effects develop when bromocriptine and levodopa are used together, one of the drugs must be reduced. If the patient has suffered with motor fluctuations that are improved after the addition of bromocriptine, we reduce the levodopa dose when toxic side effects develop, and attempt to maintain the bromocriptine at the present level. Because the plasma half-life of levodopa is shorter than that of bromocriptine, acute toxicity can often be reversed quickly by reducing levodopa. If bromocriptine is to be stopped, it can be discontinued without weaning. Nausea and vomiting occur with bromocriptine and can be controlled with the use of domperidone; additional carbidopa will not abate this effect.

PERGOLIDE

Efficacy

Pergolide was developed as a second ergot preparation to treat Parkinson's disease. It is 10 times more potent than bromocriptine, and the usual total daily dose is 1-4 mg. Like bromocriptine, pergolide has been studied as an adjunct to levodopa or Sinemet, and has significantly abated parkinsonian disability in patients with advanced Parkinson's disease. Kurlan et al. [9] studied 11 patients all with advanced (Stage IV) disease, and demonstrated a 68% increase in mobile "on" time. Like bromocriptine, however, improvement was not indefinitely maintained, and by 6 months the improvement was only 30%; improvement had disappeared by 18 months. They found that partial but temporary restoration of mobility was achieved by switching some patients to alternate-day therapy with pergolide and to daily therapy with levodopa. Similarly, in 17 patients with advanced Parkinson's disease studied for at least 2 years, Lieberman et al. [12] reported that patient initially responded with 60% group improvement in global disability. By 2 years, although still 20% less disabled than at study entry, patients found that the effect of pergolide had significantly waned. Similar patterns of improvement with pergolide have been reported by our group and others [3,4,17].

We [3] studied 22 patients for 1 year, and showed statistically significant improvement in global disability and gait difficulties with pergolide; maximal improvement was seen at 6 months and then waned slightly. No added improvement was seen, in spite of dosage adjustment, after 6 months of therapy. In those patients with motor fluctuations, improvement was maintained for the full year and, in 2 patients, the problem resolved. No patient developed new motor fluctuations while receiving pergolide. Jankovic [6] found even after 2 years that the amount of mobile "on" time remained 63% greater than before pergolide. These studies together demonstrate the efficacy of pergolide; although it does not have eternal efficacy, its capacity to reverse clinical disability for as long as 2 years in a continually progressive illness marks pergolide as a significant potential addition to antiparkinsonian therapies.

Toxicity

Like bromocriptine, pergolide is associated with side effects that are similar in frequency and type to those of bromocriptine [4]. Early in the study of pergolide, questions of cardiac toxicity were raised and this point has delayed its more widespread use and availability. To settle this controversy, Tanner et al. [16] administered pergolide for 1 year to 6 patients with stable heart disease, and monitored their neurologic and cardiac disabilities. Parkinson's disease improved in all patients, and cardiac status never worsened. They concluded that pergolide is a safe and effective therapy for parkinsonian patients, even when they have stable cardiac disease. The other systemic side effects of pergolide are similar to those seen with bromocriptine therapy. Hepatotoxicity and pleural thickening should be regarded as potential side effects of this drug. Neurologic side effects include chorea, dystonia, and myoclonus, and these abate with lower doses of the drug. Mental changes including agitation, depression, insomnia, hallucinations, and psychotic behavior may occur early in therapy or after several months. Stern and colleagues [15] specifically studied neurobehavioral deficits in patients before and while receiving chronic pergolide and found no significant change in mental abnormalities related to pergolide.

Practical Recommendations

We begin pergolide with a trial dose of 0.1 mg and increase the dose to approximately 1.0 mg/day after 2-4 weeks. The same procedure as that outlined with bromocriptine introduction is recommended. Most patients with advanced Parkinson's disease will require 2-5 mg/day in three, four, or more divided doses. As with bromocriptine, therapeutic effects of pergolide may lag behind the increase in dose by several days, so we do not recommend changing the dose more rapidly than once weekly. Similarly, when toxic effects develop with pergolide and the dose is reduced, the adverse reaction may persist for several days. In most cases where patients have motor fluctuations that have been reduced with pergolide, we try to manage central side effects such as chorea or hallucinations by first reducing the levodopa dose and maintaining the pergolide. Often the adverse reaction will clear sufficiently within 48 hours and permit a stabilization of the patient without necessitating any change in the pergolide dose. If pergolide is to be stopped, there is no withdrawal syndrome, so gradual weaning is not necessary.

COMPARATIVE STUDIES OF BROMOCRIPTINE AND PERGOLIDE

It is of clinical and economic importance to know whether one of these two agents is in fact superior to the other. Only a few studies have specifically addressed the relative safety and efficacy of bromocriptine and pergolide. Because bromocriptine was available several years before pergolide, most patients who have received both drugs received bromocriptine first—when they were younger and when their disease was less advanced. In a short-term study, LeWitt et al. [11] compared the two drugs in 9 patients with mild parkinsonism and in 15 with advanced disease in a double-blind crossover study; they found that the two drugs were equivalent and they could not favor one over the other for efficacy or side-effect profile. Lieberman et al. [14] treated 25 patients chronically with bromocriptine, then with pergolide. They favored pergolide, because it maintained its efficacy longer than bromocriptine, even though the pergolide was used later in the disease course. Goetz et al. [4] conducted a 5-year study in which 10 patients who initially responded to bromocriptine remained on this drug until efficacy waned (mean 29 months); they then switched to pergolide and were followed for a total study duration of 5 years. Three conclusions were made:

1. After 5 years of agonist therapy in addition to levodopa, patients were improved compared to the disability at study entry.
2. Although peak efficacy was equivalent between the two drugs, pergolide remained effective longer than bromocriptine in these patients.
3. In spite of having failed to continue responding to bromocriptine, these patients all promptly responded to a second agonist.

This last observation suggests that all agonists are not identical and offers hope to patients whose response to one agonist has waned. Whether the patients who switched to pergolide and had improved efficacy will be able to again return to bromocriptine with renewed drug responsiveness has yet to be studied.

FUTURE PERSPECTIVES

The identification of different types of dopamine receptors, depending on their linkage to enzymes or their anatomic location, offers the biochemist the opportunity to design agonists to stimulate one population preferentially. Future drugs that will stimulate only D-2 receptors without activating other subtypes could enhance the efficacy and also diminish the likelihood of toxic side effects. The observation that at least 4 agonists with antiparkinsonian efficacy were developed but later abandoned because of toxicity demonstrates that specificity and selectivity of these drugs is still not highly developed.

REFERENCES

1. Caraceni T, Giovannini P, Parati E, Scigliano G, Grassi MP, Carella F: Bromocriptine and lisuride in Parkinson's disease. Adv Neurol 40:531-535, 1984.
2. Glantz RH, Goetz CG, Nausieda PA, Weiner WJ, Klawans HL: The effect of bromocriptine on the on-off phenomenon. J Neural Trans 52:41-47, 1981.
3. Goetz CG, Tanner CM, Glantz RH, Klawans HL: Pergolide in Parkinson's disease. Arch Neurol 40:785-787,1983.
4. Goetz CG, Tanner CM, Glantz RH, Klawans HL: Chronic agonist therapy for Parkinson's disease: a five year study of bromocriptine and pergolide. Neurology 35:749-751, 1985.
5. Hoehn MM, Elton RL: Low dosages of bromocriptine added to levodopa in Parkinson's disease. Neurology 35:199-206, 1985.
6. Jankovic J: Long-term study of pergolide in parkinson's disease. Neurology 35:296-299, 1985.
7. Kartzinel R, Perlow M, Teychenne P: Bromocriptine and levodopa in Parkinsonism. Lancet 2:473-476, 1975.
8. Kartzinel R, Shoulson I, Calne DB: Studies with bromocriptine: double-blind comparison with levodopa in idiopathic parkinsonism. Neurology 26:511-513, 1976.
9. Kurlan R, Miller C, Levy R, Macik B, Hamill R, Shoulson I: Long-term experience with pergolide therapy of advanced parkinsonism. Neurology 35:738-742, 1985.
10. Larsen TA, Newman R, LeWitt P, Calne DB: Severity of Parkinson's disease and the dosage of bromocriptine. Neurology 34:795-797, 1984.
11. LeWitt PA, Ward CD, Larsen TA, Raphaelson MI, Newman RP, Foster N, Dambrosiam JM, Calne DB: Comparison of pergolide and bromocriptine therapy in parkinsonism. Neurology 33:1009-1014, 1983.
12. Lieberman AN, Goldstein M, Liebowitz M, Gopinathan G, Neophytides A, Hiesiger E, Nelson J, Walker R: Long-term effects of pergolide. Neurology 33(Suppl 2):112, 1983.
13. Lieberman AN, Kupersmith M, Casson I, Durso R, Foo SH, Khayali M, Tartaro T, Goldstein M: Bromocriptine and lergotrile: comparative efficacy in Parkinson's disease. Adv Neurol 24:461-473, 1979.
14. Lieberman AN, Neophytides A, Leibowitz M, Gopinathan G, Pact V, Walker R, Goodgold A, Goldstein M: Comparative efficacy of pergolide and bromocriptine in patients with advanced Parkinson's disease. Adv Neurol 37:95-108, 1983.
15. Stern Y, Mayeux R, Ilson J, Fahn S, Cote L: Pergolide therapy for Parkinson's disease: Neurobehavioral changes. Neurology 34:201-204, 1984.

16. Tanner CM, Chhablani R, Goetz CG, Klawans HL: Pergolide mesylate: lack of cardiac toxicity in patients with cardiac disease. Neurology 35:918-921, 1985.

17. Tanner CM, Goetz CG, Glantz RH, Glatt SL, Klawans HL: Pergolide mesylate and idiopathic Parkinson disease. Neurology 32:1175-1179, 1982.

Chapter 9

Recognition and Management of Major Behavior Problems in Parkinson's Disease*

Karen Marder and Richard Mayeux**

THE INTRODUCTION OF LEVODOPA IN THE LATE 1960S required physicians treating Parkinson's disease (PD) to distinguish between disease-related mental changes and those induced by medications. The goal of this chapter is to describe the characteristics of these changes and address important aspects of practical management.

DEPRESSION

Depression is the most common primary psychiatric disorder in PD. The association of PD with depression was first noted by James Parkinson in his classic essay on the Shaking Palsy in 1817. However, subsequent debate has involved three main issues: 1) the relationship of depression to disease severity and duration; 2) whether depression is endogenous or a reaction to chronic disability; 3) whether the depression is related to various treatments. The third point would seem unlikely because the presence of depression in PD was noted prior to the advent of modern therapy for PD, including levodopa.

It is important to adhere to strict definitions of depression, not only because the literature in the past has been so confusing, but also because

---

* This work is from the departments of Neurology and Psychiatry, College of Physicians and Surgeons, Columbia University. It was supported by a Health Services grant AG 02802.

** Correspondence should be addressed to Dr. Richard Mayeux, Neurological Institute, 710 West 168th Street, New York, New York 10032.

parkinsonian depression may be difficult to diagnose. Major depression syndrome and dysthymic disorder, defined in the *Third Edition of the Diagnostic and Statistical Manual of Mental Disorders (DSM III)*, are the two most common depressive disorders. Depression occurs in the absence of an organic mental syndrome or alteration in consciousness [11]. Vogel [53] suggests that parkinsonian depression is complex, but discernable, if more elementary dysfunctions are considered. For example, he suggests: 1) that psychomotor retardation occurs both in PD and depression; 2) that dementia occurring with depression may result in slowness of thinking and in disorders of concentration; and 3) that hypomimia and hypophonia might be interpreted as signs of depressed mood if self-rating scales are not used. Parkinsonians without depression experience vegetative signs such as anorexia, fatigue, insomnia, and decreased concentration. For these reasons, strict adherence to the diagnostic criteria mentioned above can be very useful.

In 1967, Warburton conducted one of the first large-scale prospective investigations of depression in PD by comparing parkinsonians with patients who had medical and surgical disorders. Parkinsonians were found to be significantly more depressed (52% of men, 60% women; control men 1%, control women 11%); no relationship between the depressive symptoms and age, duration, and severity of the illness could be established. He concluded that depression in PD must be a reaction to the disease process rather than an integral part of the disease itself [55].

Mindham [34] also concluded that the depression in PD was a reaction to disability, noting that only 12% were depressed prior to the onset of motor impairment. He further acknowledged that mood might improve independent of improvement in physical condition and advocated trials of antidepressants.

The Hamilton Depression Rating Scale (HDRS) was used retrospectively to review a series of parkinsonian patients seen over a 15-year period by Brown; 52% were depressed [5]. The correlation of rigidity and depression suggested a possible neurochemical link between motor and mental symptoms. To determine whether depression in Parkinson's disease was merely a reaction to a chronic disabling disease, Horn [14] and Robins [42] compared a group of parkinsonians with an age-matched group of physically disabled controls. Using the depression scales from the Minnesota Multiphasic Personality Index (MMPI) and the HDRS, both investigators found that depressive symptoms in PD were related to the illness, independent of its severity.

Excluding Mindham's study, where an unusually high prevalence of depression was found in parkinsonian patients admitted to a psychiatric facility, most studies using acceptable criteria and methods of investigation indicate that 40-50% of patients will experience depression. The question of whether the mood changes are reactive or are inherent remains unanswered.

The presence of depression prior to the onset of the motor symptoms supports the view that depression is endogenous. Patrick and Levy in 1922 found 34% patients were depressed prior to the onset of motor manifestations [37], and Mayeux et al. in 1981 [27] found that 25% of their depressed parkinsonians had met *DSM III* criteria for a depressive episode prior to other symptoms. Many patients also become depressed immediately or within a year of the onset of the motor manifestations of PD.

Treatment of depression has met with variable success. Tricyclic antidepressants, electroconvulsive therapy (ECT), bromocriptine, and experimental medications have been tried alone or in addition to medications used to ameliorate the motor symptoms of Parkinson's disease. It is important to recognize that failure with one mediation does not preclude a successful response to a different treatment modality.

Beginning in 1959, tricyclic antidepressants were evaluated in depressed patients with PD. Sigwald et al. [46] found that 75% of patients treated with imipramine 100-400 mg/day were improved in both mood and motor symptoms, especially akinesia. Latinen [17] subsequently performed a double-blind placebo-controlled trial of desipramine in 39 patients, and found that 63% of the patients in the desipramine group showed an overall improvement in signs and symptoms of PD compared with 16% of the placebo group. Nine of the 10 patients in the desipramine group who showed good overall improvement were less depressed and fatigued. Similarly, Andersen et al. [2] studied parkinsonians with depression who were treated optimally with levodopa using a double-blind crossover study to compare nortriptyline and placebo (50-150 mg/day). After 16 weeks, neurological signs remained unchanged, but the median depression score was significantly reduced in patients treated with nortriptyline.

Prior to the use of levodopa, parkinsonian patients given tricyclic antidepressants improved neurologically, particularly in rigidity and akinesia. The beneficial effects of tricyclics are thought to be due to their abilities to increase serotonergic and noradrenergic activity rather than to a central anticholingeric effect, which might not be apparent measuring motor signs of patients already on levodopa. Imipramine and desipramine, have less anticholinergic activity than amitryptyline and may be better tolerated in the elderly or those patients with dementia.

Several reports suggest that ECT may relieve depression in PD, even when tricyclic antidepressants are no longer effective. Lebensohn and Jenkins reported improvement in both motor and depressive symptoms in two patients after 4 treatments of ECT [18]. They suggested that ECT may increase the synthesis of dopamine and norepinephrine, or increase dopamine receptor sensitivity. Improvement in extrapyramidal function was apparent after ECT, and depression was improved later in one patient reported by Asnis [3]. He concluded that the duration of biochemical changes after ECT had not been systematically studied. Transient improvement was also found by Brown [6] in 7 patients with more severe depression. These patients were also demented.

Bromocriptine, a dopamine agonist, has recently been compared to imipramine under double-blind conditions in depressed patients [54]. The two drugs produced equal improvement in symptoms. Jouvent et al. [16] used 2.5-30 mg/day of bromocriptine for 8 days, in 10 patients with PD and depression. A good correlation between improvement in antidepressant and antiparkinsonian effects in 9 out of 10 patients were seen.

Recently it has been suggested that depressed parkinsonians may have reduced brain content of serotonin because CSF 5-HIAA (the major metabolite of serotonin) was lower in depressed patients [30]. In a pilot study, 5-HTP, the serotonin precursor, showed some benefit in depressed patients [32].

DRUG-RELATED MENTAL CHANGES

All the medications used in the treatment of Parkinson's disease are known to cause psychiatric disturbances, especially in those patients who have preexisting intellectual impairment. These psychiatric complications include delirium and hallucinations. Delirium, as defined in the *DSM III,* is characterized by a clouding of consciousness, and at least two of the following: perceptual disturbance (illusions or hallucinations), incoherent speech, insomnia or drowsiness, or increased or decreased psychomotor activity. There is also disorientation, memory impairment, and fluctuation in course.

Some patients will experience vivid visual hallucinations during treatment with antiparkinsonian medication. Insight is generally preserved, and the patient does not meet criteria for dementia or delirium. This phenomenon has been called *benign hallucinosis,* which can be relieved by reduction in anticholinergics or dopaminergic drugs.

Levodopa

Psychiatric disorders are well recognized complications of levodopa, and occur in approximately one third of patients during the course of levodopa treatment. Symptoms generally resolve quickly when levodopa is decreased or discontinued. Damasio et al. [9] noted that the onset of insomnia and anxiety can be considered a prodrome of acute psychosis.

Celesia et al. [8] administered up to 8 grams of levodopa daily to 45 patients. Psychiatric phenomena developed in 35.5% of their patients, half of whom developed frank psychosis with delusions, hallucinations, and impaired memory and orientation. Four of 6 patients who developed an associated confusional state had an underlying mild chronic organic brain syndrome. The mean latency between onset of treatment and the beginning of the psychosis was 4 months. Other psychiatric phenomena observed included euphoria and acute anxiety, both of which seemed to be related to the dose of levodopa. There was a frequent association of involuntary dyskinetic movement and psychic disturbances.

These findings were confirmed by Goodwin [13]. They noted that rapidly increasing the dosage of antiparkinsonian medication was related to these adverse effects, particularly in patients with dementia.

Rondot et al. [43] found hallucinations, confusion, and delirium in 21% of 400 patients. In one third of the cases, the onset of the confusional syndrome was related to a change in treatment. Anxiety was observed in 10% of cases and occurred acutely in some patients. Reducing or discontinuing levodopa frequently improved anxiety.

Psychiatric complications are among the most serious side effects of levodopa, and are often the reason for reduction in dosage or withdrawal of medication [20]. Goetz et al. [12] studied hallucinations in parkinsonians. Three groups were identified—one group with onset or exacerbation of symptoms related to an increase in the dose of dopaminergic medication, one group with hallucinations related to an increase in anticholinergic medication, and one group with symptoms unrelated to changes in medication. Hallucinations associated with dopaminergic agents are classically described as including a sense of heightened awareness of objects, forms, and colors superimposed on a clear sensorium, as well as hypnogogic phenomena. At very high doses, de novo hallucinatory experiences may occur. Hallucinations associated with long-term levodopa treatment usually occur in the presence of a clear sensorium and are relatively consistent among all patients. Viscual hallucinations are usual, and consist of formed images of sedentary people or animals, sometimes threatening. Auditory hallucinations are rare but can mimic schizophreniform symptoms. The character of the hallucinations for any given patient seems to be consistent regardless of which drugs are used. Decreasing the dosage of either levodopa or anticholinergic medications may reduce hallucinations. Goetz et al. [12] suggests a common pathophysiologic mechanism triggered by manipulation of neurotransmitters.

Other psychiatric disorders have been associated with levodopa use, including hypomania (almost always experienced when patients with prior history of mania are challenged with the drug), impulsivity, increased anxiety, insomnia, vivid dreams, and hypersexuality [50].

Nausieda et al. [35] found sleep complaints beginning after the onset of Parkinson's disease in 74 out of 100 consecutive patients in a Parkinson's disease clinic. Sleep-related complaints increased in proportion to the duration of levodopa treatment, but were not related to duration of therapy. Sleep fragmentation, which includes insomnia at night and excessive daytime sleepiness, is the most frequently reported complaint. Altered dreams and nocturnal vocalizations are related symptoms. Paulson et al. [38] suggested that avoiding excessive medication at bedtime may be helpful. Occasionally, the use of L-tryptophan, 500 mg before bedtime, will diminish restless sleep and vivid dreams.

Hypersexuality has been reported in patients receiving levodopa, often occurring in association with other symptoms suggestive or hypomania such as grandiosity, hyperactivity, and euphoria. O'Brien et al. [36] noted the return of spontaneous erections in 6 of 9 patients after levodopa treatment, although return of sexual interest usually parallels improvement in general motor function.

Anticholinergics

Anticholinergic agents, like levodopa, are more likely to cause confusion in the elderly and demented. DeSmet et al. [10] observed confusional states in 93% of demented parkinsonians receiving anticholinergic agents compared with 46% of the demented patients not receiving anticholinergics. Disappearance of confusion occurred after discontinuation of medication. Mental impairment and delirium can result from anticholinergics in the absence of dementia. When hallucinations occur, they are classically associated with delirium and prominent peripheral autonomic effects. Visual halluncinations are usually poorly formed and frightening.

Pergolide

Pergolide is a dopamine agonist that may cause the gamut of behavioral changes seen with levodopa, including confusion, delirium, hallucinations, anxiety, and altered sexual behavior. These symptoms remit spontaneously or disappear with reduction of dosage. Stern et al. [48] studied 19 parkinsonian patients with a full neuropsychological battery, before and after treatment with pergolide. They found that, like levodopa, patients with previous psychiatric symptoms were more prone to experience a recurrence of symptoms on low doses of pergolide. If patients had hallucinations on other medications, they were likely to do so on pergolide.

Bromocriptine/Lergotrile

Bromocriptine and lergotrile are also more likely to produce confusional symptoms in patients with an antecedent organic mental syndrome and in older patients. In a study by Serby et al. [45], 17 of 66 patients on bromocriptine and 14 of 53 patients on lergotrile developed mental changes.

DEMENTIA

Parkinsonian patients become demented more frequently than do healthy adults of similar age. Boller et al. [4] and others [21,31] suggest that there is an increased risk of dementia in patients with PD. However, the actual prevalence of dementia in any cohort of patients with PD is currently a course of controversy [7]. Prevalence estimates of dementia vary because of serious sampling problems and the failure to utilize acceptable criteria for diagnosis. The reported figures range from 15% to 30% [23,24,28], although 90% has also been cited [40]. Conversely, using currently accepted criteria for dementia, such as that of *DSM III*, recent studies indicate a prevalence of 10% to 15% [31,7,19,51]. The adjusted estimated risk of developing dementia in PD may be 3 to 5 times greater than that expected for healthy adults, depending on the age of onset of the motor manifestations [31].

The dementia of PD, when defined by uniform criteria or as a global impairment of intellectual function, is clinically and biologically similar to Alzheimer's disease. Although this is controversial, there are several lines of evidence pointing to an association between Parkinson's disease and Alzheimer's disease:

1. Dementia, once present, is clinically indistinguishable from Alzheimer's disease and similar disorders [29].
2. Pathological features of Alzheimer's disease (e.g., neurofibrillary tangles and senile plaques) are present in nearly one half of patients with Parkinson's diease, many of whom are demented [1]. In one study, the degree of tangle and plaque formation correlated with the severity of dementia in patients with PD [4].
3. The biochemical alterations of Alzheimer's disease are also present in demented patients with PD [44]. However, a reduction in brain choline acetyltransferase (CAT), the rate-limiting enzyme in the production of acetylcholine, may be present in parkinsonian brains with or without coincident pathological features of Alzheimer's disease [39].
4. The basal forebrain, an area of interest in Alzheimer's disease because of its cholinergic properties, is also subject to cell loss in parkinsonian patients with dementia [56].

Drugs and Dementia

Anticholinergics no doubt contribute to serious management problems in demented patients with PD. DeSmet and associates [10] believe that confusion, delirium, and drug-induced hallucinations are more often seen in patients (with or without dementia) when taking anticholinergics. They found that demented parkinsonians were more likely to experience these drug-induced problems when receiving anticholinergic medications. These observations are supported by the studies of CAT activity in demented parkinsonian patients because anticholinergics would further compromise the failing cholinergic system, although there is no evidence that anticholinergic medications produce a permanent dementia.

Medications with anticholinergic properties such as tricyclic antidepressants should be avoided in demented patients with PD. Similarly, peripheral-acting anticholinergics used for bladder control may precipitate confusion or delirium, because at high concentrations they may cross the blood-brain barrier. We therefore suggest that all medications with anticholinergic properties be avoided in patients with dementia.

The use of levodopa in parkinsonian patients with dementia is also challenging. Even though levodopa is usually well tolerated early in the course of disease, dementia and related problems often affect drug tolerance as the disease evolves [20]. It has been suggested that levodopa might even contribute to the development of dementia, but this is unproven and may in part be a reflection of the more normal life span of levodopa-treated patients [11]. Levodopa, as with other medications, can result in drug-induced delirium and hallucinations. Withdrawal of this agent often improves mentation dramatically. However, there is often a return to the pre-levodopa parkinsonian motor state. Other dopamine agonists such as bromocriptine, pergolide, and lisuride are all capable of inducing hallucinations and delirium, particularly in demented patients (see above).

No therapeutic agents have been found to treat the dementia of PD. Lecithin reportedly showed slight improvement [52], but this has not been confirmed. Currently, other pharmacotherapeutic agents are under investigation for the treatment of dementia.

OTHER FORMS OF INTELLECTUAL IMPAIRMENT

Other than dementia, as we have defined it, a number of unique and interesting intellectual deficits occur in patients with PD. These include bradyphrenia, visuospatial deficits, tip-of-the-tongue phenomenon, and executive-function disorders.

Bradyphrenia, defined as a disorder of attention and vigilance, is accompanied by an impairment of general intellect that is similar to that seen in mild Alzheimer's disease. However, the attenion deficit is peculiar to parkinsonians. It is characterized by a general slowing of intellect, and may be manifest in daily tasks requiring sustained attention. No treatment has been identified, but noradrenergic agonists might be considered, because increased turnover of norepinephrine may be the biochemical deficit [33].

Visuospatial deficits disrupt predictive movements, and may result from dopamine loss and basal ganglia dysfunction, unique to PD [47]. This is usually observed in neuropsychological tasks requiring drawing or copying designs. Visuospatial deficits appear in patients with MPTP-induced parkinsonism, which is considered a purely dopamine-deficiency syndrome [49]. In addition, Matthews and Haaland [26] suggest that visuospatial deficits progress with the duration of illness, whereas Loranger et al. [22] claim that cognition improves, at least transiently, on levodopa. However, the long-term effects of levodopa on mental functioning in PD remains a complex and controvesial subject requiring further investigation.

Executive-function disorder, defined as impairment of mental set-classing or sequencing behavior, is considered by some to be a frontal lobe disorder, and has been observed in patients with PD. Stern and Langston [49] found this syndrome in patients with MPTP-induced parkinsonism, and Javoy-Agid and colleagues [15] have noted a reduction of dopamine concentrations in the frontal cortex in some parkinsonians, suggesting a possible relationship between dopamine loss and frontal lobe dysfunction.

Tip-of-the-tongue phenomena [25] may also be encountered in patients with PD, and may mimic memory loss. This is usually a word-production anomia that is resistent to pharmacological intervention. It is usually not associated with dementia.

CONCLUSION

The management of behavioral problems in PD depends on correct diagnosis. This chapter provides guidelines to diagnosis and suggestions for successful intervention. It is important to remember that successful treatment of PD depends upon the recognition and management of concomitant behavioral problems.

REFERENCES

1. Alvord EC, Forno LS, Kusske JA, Kauffman RJ, Rhodes JS, Goetowski CR: The pathology of parkinsonism: A comparison of degenerations in cerebral cortex and brainstem. Adv Neurol 5:175-193, 1975.
2. Anderson J, Aabro E, Gulman N, Hjelmsted A, Pedersen HE: Antidepressant treatment of Parkinson's disease. Acta Neurol Scand 62:210-221, 1982.
3. Asnis G: Parkinson's disease, depression, and ECT: a review and case study. Am J Psychiatry 134:191-195, 1977.
4. Boller F, Mizutani T, Roessman U, Gambetti P: Parkinson's disease, dementia and Alzheimer's disease: clinopathological correlations. Ann Neurol 1:329-335, 1980.
5. Brown GL: Parkinsonism and depression. South Med J 65:540-545, 1967.
6. Brown GL: Parkinsonism, depression and ECT. Am J Psychiat 132:1084, 1975.
7. Brown RG, Marsden CD: How common is dementia in Parkinson's disease? Lancet 1:1262-1265, 1984.
8. Celesia G, Barr A: Psychosis and other psychiatric manifestations of levodopa therapy. Arch Neurol 23:193-200, 1970.
9. Damasio A, Lobo-Antunes J, Macedo C: Psychiatric aspects in parkinsonism treated with L-dopa. J Neurol Neurosurg Psychiat 34: 502-507, 1971.
10. DeSmet Y, Ruberg M, Serdana M, Dubois B, Lhermitte F, Agid Y: Confusion, dementia and anticholinergics in Parkinson's diease. J Neurol Neurosurg Psychiat 45:1161-1164, 1982.
11. Diagnostic and Statistical Manual of Mental Disorders (3rd ed). Washington, DC, American Psychiatric Association, 1980.

12. Goetz C, Tanner C, Klawans H: Pharmacology of hallucinations induced by long-term drug therapy. Am J Psychiat 139:494-497, 1982.
13. Goodwin FK: Psychiatric side effects of levodopa in man. JAMA 218:1915-1920, 1979.
14. Horn S: Some psychological factors in parkinsonism. J Neurol Neurosurg Psychiatr 37:27-31, 1974.
15. Javoy-Agid F, Agid Y: Is the mesocortical dopaminergic system involved in Parkinson's disease? Neurology 30:1326-1330, 1980.
16. Jouvent R, Abensour P, Bonnet A, Wedlocher D, Lhermitte F, Agid Y: Antiparkinsonian and antidepressant effects of high doses of bromocriptine: independent comparison of neurologic and psychiatric effects. J Affect Disord 2:141-145, 1983.
17. Laitinen L: Desipramine in the treatment of Parkinson's disease. Acta Neurol Scand 45:109-113, 1969.
18. Lebensohn Z, Jenkins RB: Improvement of parkinsonism in depressed patients with ECT. Am J Psychiat 132:283-285, 1975.
19. Lees AJ: Parkinson's disease and dementia. Lancet 1:43-44, 1985.
20. Lesser RP, Fahn S, Snider SR, Cote LJ, Isgreen WP, Barrett RE: Analysis of the clinical problems in parkinsonism and the complications of long-term levodopa therapy. Neurology 20:1253-1260, 1979.
21. Lieberman A, Dziatolowski M, Coopersmith M, Cerb M, Goodgold A, Orcin J, Goldstein M: Dementia in Parkinson's disease. Ann Neurol 6:335-359, 1979.
22. Loranger AW, Goodell H, Lee JE, McDowell F: Levodopa treatment of Parkinson's syndrome. Arch Gen Psychiat 26:163-168, 1972.
23. Martin WE, Loewenson RB, Resch JA, Baker AB: Parkinson's disease: clinical analysis of 100 patients. Neurology 23:783-790, 1973.
24. Martilla RJ, Rinne UK: Dementia in Parkinson's disease. Acta Neur Scand 54:431-441, 1976.
25. Matison R, Mayeux R, Rosen J, Fahn S: "Tip-of-the-tongue" phenomenon in Parkinson's disease. Neurology 32:567-570, 1982.
26. Matthews CG, Haaland KY: The effect of symptom duration on cognitive and motor performance in parkinsonism. Neurology 29:951-956, 1979.
27. Mayeux R, Stern Y, Rosen J, Leventhal J: Depression, intellectual impairment and Parkinsons disease. Neurology 31:645-650, 1981.
28. Mayeux R: Depression and dementia in Parkinson's disease. In Marsden CD, Fahn S (eds): Movement Disorders. London, Butterworth pp 75-95, 1982.
29. Mayeux R, Stern Y, Rosen J, Benson F: Subcortical dementia: a recognizable clinical entity. Ann Neurol 14:278-283, 1983.
30. Mayeux R, Stern Y, Cote L, Williams JBW: Altered serotonin metabolism in depressed patients with Parkinson's disease. Neurology 34:642-646, 1984.
31. Mayeux R, Rosenstein R, Stern Y, Cote L, Fahn S: The prevalence and risk of dementia in idiopathic Parkinson's disease. Arch Neurol 45:260-262, 1988.
32. Mayeux R, Stern Y, Sano M, Williams J, Cote L: The relationship of serotonin to depression in Parkinson's disease. Ann Neurol 20:149, 1986.
33. Mayeux R, Stern Y, Sano M, Cote L, Williams JBM: Clinical and biochemical correlates of bradyphrenia in Parkinson disease. Neurology 37:1130-1134, 1987.

34. Mindham RHS, Marsden CD, Parkes JD: Psychiatric symptoms during L-dopa therapy for Parkinson's disease and their relationship to physical disability. Psychiatr Med 6:23-33, 1967.

35. Nausieda P, Glanz R, Weber S, Baum R, Klawans HL: Psychiatric complications of levodopa therapy of Parkinson's disease. In Hassler RG, Christ JF (eds): Parkinson-specific Motor and Mental Disorders. New York, Raven Press, pp 271-278, 1984.

36. O'Brien C, DiGiacomo JN, Fahn S, Schwartz GA: Mental effects of high dosage levedopa. Arch Gen Psychiat 24:61-64, 1971.

37. Patrick HT, Levy D: Parkinson's disease: a clinical study of 146 cases. Arch Neurol Psychiat 7:711-720, 1922.

38. Paulson G, Schafer K, Hallum B: Avoiding mental changes and falls in older Parkinson's patients. Geriatrics 41:59-62, 1986.

39. Perry RH, Tomlinson BE, Candy JM, Blessed G, Foster JF, Bloxham CA, Perry E: Cortical cholinergic deficit in mentally impaired parkinsonian patients. Lancet 2: 789-790, 1983.

40. Pirozzolo FJ, Hansch EC, Mortimer JA, Webster DD, Kuskowski MA: Dementia in Parkinson's disease: a neuropsychological analysis. Brain Cognition 1:71-83, 1982.

41. Rajput AH, Offord K, Beard CM, Kurland LT: Epidemiological survey of dementia in parkinsonism and a control population. Adv Neurol 40:229-234, 1984.

42. Robins AH: Depression in patients with parkinsonism. Br J Psychiat 128:141-145, 1976.

43. Rondot P, deRecondo J, Coignet A, Ziegler M: Mental Disorders in Parkinson's disease. In Hassler RG, Christ J (eds): Parkinson- specific Motor and Mental disorders. New York, Raven Press, 1984.

44. Ruberg M, Ploska A, Javoy-Agid F, Agid Y: Muscarinic binding and choline acetyltransferase activity in parkinsonian subjects with reference to dementia. Brain Res 232:129-133, 1982.

45. Serby M, Angrist B, Lieberman A: Mental disturbances during bromocriptine and lergotrile treatment of Parkinson's disease. Am J Psychiat 135:1227-1229, 1978.

46. Sigwald J, Boultier D, Raymondeaud I, Marquez M, Gal JC: Etude de 'action sur l'akinesie parkinsonienne de deux derives de l'imiodibenzyle:ou imipramineou 8307 RP. Presse Med 67:1697-1698, 1959.

47. Stern Y, Mayeux R, Rosen J, Ilson J: Perceptual motor dysfunction in Parkinson's disease: a deficit in sequential and predictive movement. J Neurol Neurosurg Psychiat 46:145-151, 1983.

48. Stern Y, Mayeux R, Ilson J, Fahn S, Cote L: Pergolide treatment of Parkinson's disease: neurobehavioral changes. Neurology 34:201-203, 1984.

49. Stern Y, Langston W: Intellectual changes in patients with MPTP-induced parkinsonism. Neurology 35:1506-1509, 1985.

50. Sweet R, McDowell F, Feigenson J, Lormanger M, Goodel H: Mental symptoms in Parkinson's disease during chronic treatment with levodopa. Neurology 26:305-310, 1976.

51. Taylor A, Staint-Cyr JA, Lang AE: Dementia prevalence in Parkinson's disease. Lancet 1:1037, 1985.

52. Tweedy JR, Garcia CA: Lecithin treatment of cognitively impaired parkinsons patients. Eur J Clin Invest 12:897-90, 1982.
53. Vogel HP: Symptoms of depression in Parkinson's disease. Pharmcopsychiat 15:192-196, 1982.
54. Waehrens J, Gerlach J: Bromocriptine and imipramine in endogenous depression. A double blind controlled trial in outpatients. J Affect Disord 3:193-202, 1981.
55. Warburton JW: Depressive symptoms in parkinson patients referred for thalamotomy. J Neurol Neurosurg Psychiat 30:368-370, 1967.
56. Whitehouse P, Hedreen JC, White C, DeLong M, Price DL: Basal forebrain neurons in the dementia of Parkinson's disease. Ann Neurol 13:243-248,1983.

IV
Future Considerations

Chapter 10

Whither Parkinson's Disease?

Stanley Fahn*

THE EDITORS HAVE ASKED ME TO SPECULATE on the future trends in the understanding and treatment of Parkinson's disease (PD). This task comes at an opportune time, because there is currently much ferment in new ideas on the etiology, pathogenesis, prevention, and treatment of PD. The first and only neurologic degenerative disease to be investigated with transplantation techniques is PD, and the first successful treatment of PD with autografts of the patient's adrenal medulla has already been reported [11]. Simultaneously, the largest federally funded study on PD has just been initiated, investigating the prophylactic benefit of deprenyl and tocopherol in slowing the progression of the illness. Undoubtedly these and other research activities will lead to progress. For the patient with PD, this spells hope for the future. We witnessed a therapeutic revolution in the treatment of PD two decades ago with the introduction of high-dosage levodopa [5]. Are we now on the threshold of another revolution—not only in therapy but also in prevention?

ETIOLOGY AND PATHOGENESIS

The discovery of MPTP-induced parkinsonism [10] has given support to the hypothesis that exogenous or endogenous toxin(s) may be responsible for the cellular degeneration in PD. MPTP is a leading suspect; not only does it produce degeneration of dopaminergic neurons in the substantia nigra, but it also causes the formation of Lewy bodies and

---

* Dr. Stanley Fahn, Neurological Institute, 710 West 168th Street, New York, NY 10032, U.S.A.

degeneration of the locus ceruleus in experimental elderly nonhuman primates [6], pathological changes that are characteristic of PD. This toxin has not yet been found widely in the environment. Could there be a similar, ubiquitous environmental neurotoxin? Could such a toxin be formed within the body? Again, nothing of this nature has been yet discovered.

Nigral neurons degenerate in all animal species studied as a result of aging [12] and there is a corresponding decline of striatal dopamine and the enzymes that synthesize dopamine [4]. These facts lend credence to the idea that an endogenous mechanism located within these neurons accounts for their programmed death. Cohen [3] has pointed out that dopamine itself, when metabolized by monoamine oxidase (MAO), generates one molecule of hydrogen peroxide for every molecule of dopamine metabolized. In turn, hydrogen peroxide is linked by one electron-transfer reaction to superoxide and the hydroxyl free radicals, both of which are toxic to lipids within cells and cell membranes. Thus, excessive formation or insufficient destruction of free radicals by intrinsic antioxidant scavengers could increase the risk of PD. The genesis of excess free radical production and lack of adequate scavengers is unknown. Another possibility is that the decline of nigral neurons may be more rapid in the parkinsonian-to-be than in the person not destined to develop PD. Rather, the former may have congenitally fewer nigral neurons, and thus reach the critical number of cells below which symptoms of PD will appear as the normal age-related nigral dropout progresses.

Another source of endogenous oxidation is the conversion of dopamine to neuromelanin. Graham [8] has shown that quinones are intermediate products of the conversion and can behave as oxidizing agents. Thus, dopamine is a potential source of two toxic oxidizers—quinone and free radicals—that might facilitate the death of nigral neurons.

PROPHYLACTIC THERAPY

The above hypotheses that exogenous and endogenous toxins can cause PD have led to the development of a placebo-controlled, double-blind, randomized, multi-center study to determine if deprenyl and tocopherol can slow the progression of PD if given early in the course. L-deprenyl is an inhibitor of monoamine oxidase (MAO) type B, the enzyme that oxidizes MPTP to MPP+, the toxic metabolite of MPTP. Deprenyl pretreatment prevents MPTP- induced parkinsonism in animals. Moreover, MAO-B metabolizes dopamine and other monoamines to form hydrogen peroxide, a reaction that should also be blocked by deprenyl. Thus, deprenyl would have a two-pronged pharmacological impact—preventing MPTP-parkinsonism (as it does in animal models) and reducing free radical formation from the monoamines. In support of deprenyl as a possible prophylactic agent is the report by Birkmayer et al. [2] who suggest that PD does not progress as rapidly in patients who have been receiving L-deprenyl. Tocopherol is a well-known lipid-soluble antioxidant. Preliminary studies of its use in early PD suggest that it is safe, well tolerated—and it may be slowing the progression of parkinsonism in patients under my care (Fahn, unpublished observations). However, the need for a control group requires the rigorous assessment of effiacy that can only be accomplished through a randomized double-blind study design.

The large multicenter study now underway will randomize 800 subjects with mild untreated PD into four equal groups: 1) deprenyl, 2) tocopherol, 3) deprenyl and tocopherol, and 4) placebo. The study will last 5 years, after which we should know whether this approach will change the course of PD.

SPECIFIC THERAPIES

A potentially revolutionary new treatment of PD is the surgical transplantation of tissue into the brain to replace the missing transmitter, dopamine. Implants of embryonic nigral tissue to rodents and to subhuman primates can reverse some of the features of nigral degeneration in these animals [15]. Implants of adrenal medulla into the lateral ventricle of rodents were also partially effective in reversing parkinsonian features [7]. The first four attempts to transplant autografts of adrenal medulla to caudate in humans with PD were not similarly effective [1,14]. However, a different technique of embedding the grafts in the caudate adjacent to the ventricular wall and in contact with cerebrospinal fluid has been clinically successful, according to investigators from Mexico City [11]. This success is stimulating centers in the U.S. to attempt to reproduce the results. Madrazo (personal communication) is advocating the procedure only in patients with severe PD and who are younger than age 60. It would appear that the success of Madrazo et al. probably does not reflect the simple placement of a dopamine-generating tissue in the affected regions. Clinical benefit was seen bilaterally in the 2 reported cases, although the adrenal medullary tissue was implanted in the right caudate only. Rather, it has been proposed by Moore [13] that the implants may be releasing an unknown trophic factor(s), which stimulates recovery of the injured nigrostriatal system. Much work remains to be done in this field to understand what is actually happening.

SYMPTOMATIC THERAPIES

The most common approach in current research for PD is in the development of more effective symptomatic therapies. Most of the effort is directed at new dopaminergic drugs with a longer biological half-life to treat the all-too-common problem of clinical fluctuations seen with chronic levodopa therapy. These drugs are taking the form of sustained-release preparations of Sinemet and of Madopar. In addition, newer direct-acting dopamine agonists are being investigated. The potent agonist, 4-propyl, 9-hydroxynapthoxazine (PHNO) is promising, because it can penetrate the skin and therefore has the potential for transdermal delivery via a skin patch [9]. If this approach could maintain constant plasma and brain levels of the active agent, it is likely to become an effective treatment for clinical fluctuations.

Another approach is to determine if specific drugs could prevent the development of the complications of chronic levodopa therapy. Rinne [16] has reported that early treatment with bromocriptine has effectively reduced the occurrence of dyskinesias and fluctuations. However, his studies employed historical controls, and new prospective, randomized, controlled studies in other centers have been started to verify Rinne's findings. The concept that sustained-release Sinemet could prevent the complications seen with regular Sinemet is also being proposed. Trials to test this hypothesis may soon appear.

CONCLUSION

We are living at an exciting time in the history of knowledge and treatment of PD. Not only has this chronic neurologic disease been at the center of the pioneering demonstration of the effiacy of replacement therapy for neurotransmitter depletion (levodopa therapy), but it is also the first to be studied for the possibility of slowing progression (deprenyl and tocopherol), and the first to be the focus of tissue transplantation into the brain. If these new approaches prove to be valid, the therapeutic revolution in neurology that Cotzias and others began over 20 years ago will have taken another giant step toward better control of this and other disabling diseases of the nervous system.

REFERENCES

1. Backlund E-O, Granberg P-O, Hamberger B, Knutsson E, Martensson A, et al.: Transplantation of adrenal medullary tissue to striatum in parkinsonism. First clinical trials. J Neurosurg 62:169-173, 1985.

2. Birkmayer W, Knoll J, Riederer P. Increased life expectancy resulting from addition to L-deprenyl to Madopar treatment in Parkinson's disease: A long-term study. J Neural Transm 64:113-127, 1985.

3. Cohen G: The pathobiology of Parkinson's disease: biochemical aspects of dopamine neuron senescence. J Neural Transm 19(Suppl):89-103, 1983.

4. Cote LJ, Kremzner LT: Biochemical changes in normal aging in human brain. Adv Neurol 38:19-30, 1983.

5. Cotzias GC, Van Woert MH, Schiffer LM: Aromatic amino acids and modification of parkinsonism. N Engl J Med 276:374-379, 1967.

6. Forno LS, Langston JW, DeLanney LE, Irwin I, Ricaurte GA: Locus ceruleus lesions and eosinophilic inclusions in MPTP-treated monkeys. Ann Neurol 20:449-455, 1986.

7. Freed WJ, Morihisa JM, Spoor E, Hoffer BJ, Olson L, et al: Transplanted adrenal chromaffin cells in rat brain reduce lesion- induced rotational behavior. Nature 292:351-352, 1981.

8. Graham DG: Catecholamine toxicity: a proposal for the molecular pathogenesis of manganese neurotoxicity and Parkinson's disease. Neurotoxicol 5:83-96, 1984.

9. Grandas F, Quinn N, Critchley P, Rohan A, Marsden CD,Stahl SM: Antiparkinsonian activity of a single oral dose of PHNO. Movement Dis 2:47-51, 1987.

10. Langston JW, Ballard P, Tetrud JW, Irwin I: Chronic parkinsonism in humans due to a product of meperidine analog synthesis. Science 219:979-980, 1983.

11. Madrazo I, Drucker-Colin R, Diaz V, Martinez-Mata J, Torres C, Bercerrii JJ: Open microsurgical autograft of adrenal medulla grafts to the right caudate nucleus in two patients with intractable Parkinson's disease. N Engl J Med 316:831-834, 1987.

12. McGeer EG: Aging and neurotransmitter metabolism in the human brain. Aging 7:427-440, 1978.

13. Moore RY: Parkinson's disease: a new therapy? N Engl J Med 316:872-873, 1987.

14. Olson L, Backlund E-O, Gerhardt G, Hoffer B, Lindvall O, et al: Nigral and adrenal grafts in parkinsonism: Recent basic and clinical studies. Adv Neurol 45:85-94, 1986.

15. Perlow MJ, Freed WJ, Hoffer BJ, Seiger A, Olson L, Wyatt RJ: Brain grafts reduce motor abnormalities produced by destruction of nigrostriatal dopamine system. Science 204:643-647, 1979.

16. Rinne UK: Combined bromocriptine-levodopa therapy early in Parkinson's disease. Neurology 35:1196-1198, 1985.

Index